CHANCE ENCOUNTERS

Chance Encounters

A Bioethics for a Damaged Planet

Kristien Hens

OpenBook Publishers

https://www.openbookpublishers.com

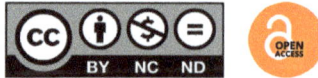

ISBN Paperback: 9781800648494
ISBN Hardback: 9781800648500
ISBN Digital (PDF): 9781800648517
ISBN Digital eBook (EPUB): 9781800648524
ISBN Digital eBook (AZW3): 9781800648531
ISBN XML: 9781800648548
ISBN HTML: 9781800648555
DOI: 10.11647/OBP.0320

Cover image: Intuitive abstract of fungal/vegetal collaborations.
Drawing by Christina Stadlbauer (2019).
Cover design by Jeevanjot Nagpal

Contents

Note to the reader regarding the choice of images and sketches

Dear reader,

The images and sketches that can be viewed in this publication were included in the following way:

By the bliss of chance, the author´s path aligned with ours — we are artists and researchers Christina Stadlbauer and Bart Vandeput (Bartaku). We both have a practice that is enquiry-based, crossing disciplines, mixing media and contexts. Kristien Hens invited us to provide visuals for her book.

We accepted, read the manuscript and observed many parallels and connections between our practice and Kristien's line of work. In particular, our frequent collaborations with scientists bring out similar questions as those voiced in the book. These enquiries drive artistic research processes and create the basis of tangible art works.

Our visual contribution provides a different angle to view the landscape Hens describes. This means that the images are not mere "illustrations" of the text but rather complement the author´s analysis. We especially hope the imagery invites you to stay joyfully with the troubles that are discussed in Kristien Hens' writings.

Thank you, Kristien, for inviting us to participate in this publication!

Prologue
Van Rensselaer Potter

In which I introduce one of the original bioethicists

The purpose of this book is to contribute to the future of the species by promoting the formation of a new discipline, the discipline of bioethics. If there are 'two cultures' that seem unable to speak to each other—science and the humanities—and if this is part of the reason that the future seems in doubt, then possible, we might build a 'bridge to the future' by building the discipline of Bioethics as a bridge between the two cultures.

—Van Rensselaer Potter (Rensselaer Potter, 1971, p. vii)

 https://doi.org/10.11647/OBP.0320.22

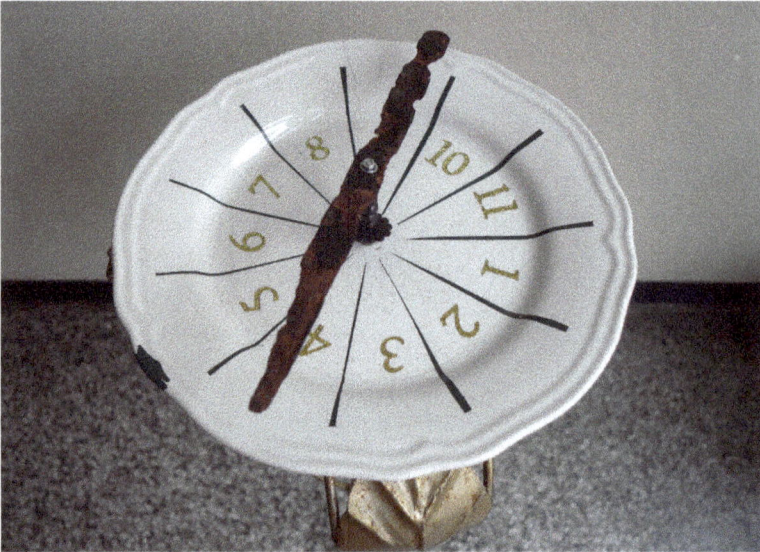

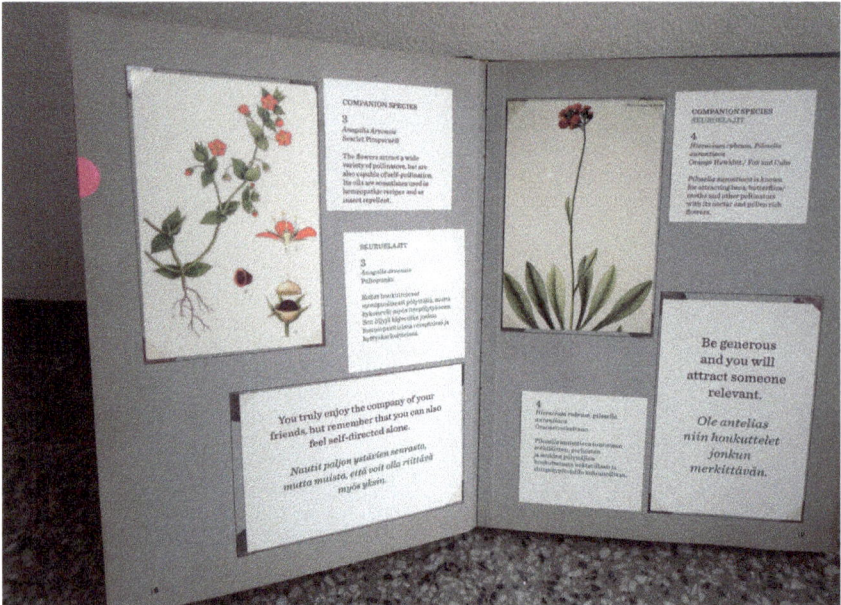

Practice to tune into time management and resilience of vegetal life forms.

From Christina Stadlbauer's The Phytonic Oracle. A tool to read into the future, based on selected plants from the FlowerClock, 2022. Photos by Christina Stadlbauer, 2022[1]

1   Christina Stadlbauer, The Phytonic Oracle; participatory installation at "Plant Measures" exhibition, Finlayson Art Area, Tampere (FI), 2022.

1. A Foundation for Bioethics

Van Rensselaer Potter's Legacy

How to live on a damaged planet? This was the question that the contributors to *Arts of Living on a Damaged Planet* asked themselves, a volume that was edited by Anna Tsing, Heather Swanson, Elaine Gan and Nils Bubandt and that appeared in 2017 (Tsing *et al.*, 2017). At the time of writing, it is 2022, and a pandemic has thrown humanity off guard. COVID-19 serves as a wake-up call for many ethicists and policymakers. How do we go forward? How to prevent, mitigate or live with even more challenging disasters yet to come? What methods do we use? What should be the guiding ethical principles? What technologies are appropriate? How will they change us? What about possible future health crises related to environmental pollution and climate change? *Bioethics* is the discipline deeply invested in questions related to technologies, health, and biology. Today, in 2022, bioethical reflections on responsibility towards future generations, our position as human animals in the biosphere, and the limitations of medicine in the face of human health crises are more needed than ever. At the same time, mainstream bioethics has still to rise fully to the occasion when facing possible future calamities.

First, bioethicists like me may have ignored the situatedness of knowledge and ethical reflection. We have assumed that a toolbox of Anglo-Saxon principles such as autonomy and beneficence (Beauchamp and Childress, 1979), or more continental ones, including dignity, would suffice in maintaining an ethical biomedical practice. We have sometimes missed opportunities to engage with other value systems and marginalized standpoints. As Henk Ten Have writes in *Bizarre Bioethics*:

   https://doi.org/10.11647/OBP.0320.01

It [bioethics] is too distanced from the values of ordinary people and too far from the social context in which problems arise. Ethics should be 'resocialized' (i.e., located into specific contexts; for example, considering the setting of poverty with the lack of access to treatment). (ten Have, 2022)

Second, our perspectives were perhaps too fringe, too easily seduced by the lure of fantastic new technologies. Maybe disproportionally too much attention has been paid to the ethics of designer babies when the world as we know it is at risk of ceasing to exist. At the same time, the challenges humanity is facing are unprecedented. As I am writing these lines, most scientists and politicians acknowledge that it will be tough to keep the global temperature rise below 1.5 degrees Celcius. It is almost certain that generations after us will face unprecedented difficulties. Bioethics has a pivotal role as health, the environment, and new technologies have been the topics of our enquiry long ago. Still, until recently, environmental or engineering ethics have played a marginal role in bioethics conferences. Questions about environmental justice and where the world should be headed are often overshadowed by discussions about genetic privacy and the risks of genetic modification. Indeed, *Arts of Living on a Damaged Planet* contains contributions of artists, writers and academics working in anthropology, history, humanities, biology, feminist philosophy, botany, ecology, literature and genetics, but no bioethicists.

Since the second half of the twentieth century, bioethics has been heavily influenced by Georgetown professors Beauchamp and Childress' book *Principles of Biomedical Ethics* (Beauchamp and Childress, 1979). This book laid down what would become the four principles of bioethics that every beginning bioethics student has to learn: autonomy, beneficence, non-maleficence, and justice. Since its publication, many have criticized it for valid reasons that will make their way into this book: the principles are too Anglo-Saxon, too Global North, too abstract and should be supplemented with situated knowledge and context-sensitive information, facts that Beauchamp and Childress themselves wholeheartedly agree with. What has not often been questioned is the task of bioethics with regard to science. Bioethics and the science it relates to are seen as two separate endeavours. Although bioethicists thinking about research ethics have thought about how to do science ethically, as in not committing fraud and protecting the privacy and integrity of research participants, we have often taken for granted the starting points and the aims of science itself. According to Henk ten Have, this has led to a reduced critical potential. As such, the agenda of bioethics accommodates 'the social and cultural context in which it has emerged' without querying the underlying values that guide science (ten Have, 2022, pp. 26–29). We do not often comment on what science there should be, what science we should want, or what future such science should create. Bioethics and exact science are seen as practices with fundamentally different methods and finalities. As if they, in the words of PC Snow, belong to *two cultures* (Snow, 1993).

Bioethics has not always been conceived as a handmaiden to science and medicine. It is worth going back into the history of 'bioethics'. One of the first people to think about ethics and science and the inseparability of health and environment was the American biochemist and professor in oncology Van Rensselaer Potter (1911–2001), as is described in Henk ten Have's book *Wounded Planet* (ten Have, 2019). Potter wrote two books: in the first, his focus was on bridging the gap between biology and ethics, and in the second, he developed a global bioethics that encompasses both societal concerns and more individual concerns, the latter being more readily associated with mainstream bioethics as we know it today. His first book *Bioethics: Bridge to the Future*, was written in 1971 (Potter, 1971). At that time, there was a need to think about a liveable future for human beings. Rachel Carson had described the potentially disastrous consequences of pesticides in her 1962 book *Silent Spring* (Carson, 2002).

Potter aimed to 'contribute to the future of human species, by promoting the formation of a new discipline, bioethics'. We now tend to forget to mention his work in bioethics courses. Potter's idea that 'ethical values cannot be separated from biological fact' is now often considered naive and potentially even dangerous. For Potter, ethics that can help us live and survive on a damaged planet should be based on biological knowledge, hence *bio*ethics. However, for him, such biological knowledge cannot be reductionist or determinist. Potter argues that the biology he thinks our knowledge should be based on is holistic, not mechanistic, as was the predominant view in the twentieth century.

Such a view of life makes it self-evident to see nature and life as objects that can be manipulated and tampered with. Biological ethics should be based on ecological and ethical holism. According to Potter, life is full of chance, feedback loops, and disorder. This disorder is the raw material for creativity, for the potential of ethical biology to imagine and create a future for humanity. We need educated leaders who are trained in both science and humanities. He describes a *Council on the Future*, quoting Margaret Mead, to use 'The future as a basis for establishing a shared culture'. Such an interdisciplinary council can function as a fourth power, independent from the legislative, executive, and judiciary powers, and needs to safeguard the future.

In his second book, *Global Bioethics*, Van Rensselaer Potter is disappointed that the bioethics he envisages has not taken flight (Potter, 1988). Instead, he writes, bioethics had become synonymous with medical ethics. According to Potter, there are two types of bioethics, medical bioethics, which has a short-term view, and environmental bioethics, with a long-term perspective. Both are part of 'global' bioethics, which considers different viewpoints, including the feminist viewpoint. His views in this book, especially his insistence on tackling overpopulation, are sometimes ableist and do not systematically consider the global south's perspectives. Still, the idea of global bioethics that extends beyond the individual relation between practitioner and patient and has a long-term view of humanity's survival as a goal is refreshing and sorely needed, especially now. So is the idea that life, science, and ethics are entangled. For Potter, ethics is based on science, as is evident from this quote: 'As concerned humans, we "ought" to consider the "is" of earth's carrying capacity and how it can be enhanced and preserved'. There may be wisdom in biology. At the same time, scientific practice should be guided by ethics and a desire to preserve humanity. Science and ethics are entangled in a non-hierarchical way.

With this book, I want to take to heart the hopes and dreams of Potter.[1] Following Potter, I argue that bioethics and biology are fundamentally entangled and show that bioethics should claim its position at the science

---

1   I am not the first to do so, see for example Henk ten Have's excellent book *Wounded Planet* (ten Have, 2019). I consider my approach complementary to his, as I will engage with posthumanist thinkers.

table from the design phase of research. Bioethics is not merely an afterthought. I also argue that bioethics can and should extend beyond medical practice or fringe cases such as genetically edited embryos and confront urgent cases such as the environmental crisis heads on. I use ideas from different thinkers, recent and less recent, that corroborate this idea. At the same time, I believe Potter's framework needs some rethinking. I have found inspiration in feminist posthumanist thinking and standpoint epistemology. Speculative bioethics, a bioethics for the future of humankind, is necessarily also an *intersectional* bioethics. It is forward-looking but not utopian and takes the trouble and messiness of the present as a starting point to develop something better. For example, I shall not follow Potter's somewhat problematic suggestion that restricting population growth is the main answer. In fact, I will not offer 'solutions' at all. I advocate for bioethics that stays with the trouble, in the words of Donna Haraway (Haraway, 2016). Quick fixes and simple solutions that strip arguments of all the ballast that may obscure them are counterproductive.

At the same time, it is not my aim to attack a 'straw man' bioethics. The book at hand is more a reflection on my readings of the last decade and a critique of my own earlier work than it aims to caricature bioethics as a field altogether. In fact, during the last decades, more and more voices have advocated for a more critical bioethics, often mentioning Potter's foundational ideas. This book is as much a description of a personal journey as it is an academic work. As I shall argue that also in bioethics, situated knowledges (and thus a critical reflection on one's own situated knowledge) matter, I think this approach is warranted. I am indebted to many great thinkers that have formulated similar ideas. For example, in her brilliant book *Bioethics in the Age of New Media*, Joanna Zylinska has pinpointed and criticized three main characteristics of 'traditional' or 'mainstream' bioethics: a sense of normativity, or being able to pinpoint what is the 'good', the rational human subject that can make a decision and is the source of this decision as a starting point, and the need for the universalization and applicability of the moral judgment (Zylinska, 2009). Zylinska offers an alternative: she is inspired by Levinas to advocate for a posthuman bioethics of 'responsibility for the infinite alterity (i.e., difference) of the other, as openness and hospitality', while at the same time offering insights from cultural and media studies. Her view on life is deeply relational:

> What we are dealing with, however, is not so much a 'human being' understood as a discrete and disembodied moral unity but rather a 'human becoming': relational, co-emerging with technology, materially implicated in sociocultural networks, and kin to other life forms (Rogers, 2022)

I will also argue for a kind of posthuman bioethics that embraces entanglements of all levels of life, although I start from different thinkers than Zylinska.

Feminist bioethicists such as Hilde Lindemann have argued for situated knowledge and the inclusion of care perspectives and understanding experiences[2] (Lindemann, 2006; Lindemann, Verkerk and Walker, 2008). Scholars such as Jackie Leach Scully and Rosemarie Garland-Thomson have convincingly argued for including a disability perspective in bioethics (Scully, 2008, 2012; Garland-Thomson, 2012).

Moreover, many colleagues have suggested that bioethics should not solely be about individual relations and responsibilities. It should question the system it operates in. These colleagues suggested that we should marry bioethics and political philosophy. For example, Joseph Millum and Ezekiel J. Emanuel argue in their volume *Global Justice and Bioethics* that bioethics must move away from parochialism:

> The facts of globalization mean that a responsible bioethics must address problems of international scope. But the expansion of the scope of both theories of justice and the problems of bioethics into the global arena means that the concerns of the two now intersect to an unprecedented degree. Consequently, it is now impossible to engage with many of the most pressing problems of bioethics without also engaging with political philosophy (if, indeed, it ever was possible) (Millum and Emanuel, 2012).

In *Global Bioethics*, Henk ten Have advocates for bioethics that acknowledges the impact of globalization on health and also questions the social, economic, and political context that is producing the problems at a global level. In *Wounded Planet* ten Have is inspired by the works

---

2   See for example the recent volume *The Routledge Handbook of Feminist Bioethics*, edited by Wendy A. Rogers, Jackie Leach Scully, Stacy M. Carter, Vikki A. Entwistle and Catherine Mills (Rogers *et al.*, 2022).

of Van Rensselaer Potter to argue for bioethics that extends beyond biomedical ethics to include environmental ethics (ten Have, 2019). In *Naturalizing Bioethics*, the editors, Hilde Lindemann, Marian Verkerk and Margaret Urban Walker, advocate for a new interpretation of naturalism in Bioethics that includes situated knowledges and analysis of power structures rather than assuming that knowledge can be produced from an Archimedean perspective:

> Our naturalism, however, does not privilege institutionally organized natural and social scientific knowledge but also embraces the experience of individuals in personal, social and institutional life. Our naturalism is also wary of idealizations that bypass social realities and of purely 'reflective' approaches to ethics that are apt to reflect only some, and usually the socially most privileged, points of view regarding the right, the good, and moral ideals such as autonomy, respect, beneficence and justice (Lindemann, Verkerk and Walker, 2008, p. 5).

In this book, I want to stand on the shoulders of these giants who have laid the foundation of rethinking bioethics to make it relevant to the challenges we are facing. In the words of Potter and Joanna Zylinska, I believe it is possible to reclaim bioethics as proper *ethics of life*. Such ethics of life includes thinking about the lives and health of humans and other-than-human beings, the macrocosmos and the entanglements of all these entities. In what follows, I investigate how to imagine bioethics as a discipline in times of superwicked problems,[3] using ideas from process philosophy, biology, and feminist posthumanism.

Such an approach implies that bioethics is a grand project that focuses on interpersonal and interspecies relations but that at the same time is political and, to use Isabelle Stengers's words, *cosmopolitical* (Stengers, 2005). The description of bioethics as a 'meeting ground', as Onora O'Neill has called it, is more than ever accurate (O'Neill, 2002). It also means that we take Van Rensselaer Potter's idea of bioethics seriously as a foundational approach permeating all scientific practice levels. Next to positioning bioethics in relation to other sciences, exact sciences, philosophy, and humanities, I also use a specific concept of life that I

---

3   Kelly Levin and colleagues described the term "super wicked" to characterize a new class of global environmental problems comprising of four key features: time is running out; those who cause the problem also seek to provide a solution; the central authority needed to address them is weak or non-existent; and irrational discounting occurs that pushes responses into the future (Levin *et al.*, 2012).

think should guide bioethics. I have borrowed this concept from systems thinkers such as Stuart Kauffman, Donna Haraway and Lynn Margulis and developmental systems theory and process philosophy. Arguing that there should be more dialogue between the sciences and bioethics and philosophy, also on very conceptual and fundamental issues, and at the same time already committing to a particular processual view on life and the universe may look contradictory. Perhaps this need not be the case. For one, process views on life offer us a way of looking at science in a way that both acknowledges the historicity of particular thought and the idea that such acknowledgement does not mean that we have to buy into the idea that everything is relative. At the same time, a new materialist or process view on matter and life also entangles ethics and science at its core. Science is as much about world-making as it is about describing the world, and describing is also world-making. Getting science right is not separated from imagining what future we want. It is at this nexus that the bioethicist is at home.

2. Overview of the Arguments

In the first part of the book, *Science*, I shall suggest a rapprochement of bioethics and the philosophy of science, specifically philosophy of biology. I shall argue that getting the concepts and the context right in science is the first ethical step for scientists. Hence, the practices of philosophers of science and bioethics are not so different, although there seems to be a wide gap between these disciplines. I will use the example of genes and a developmental approach to genes to demonstrate this. There is a place for a philosopher or ethicist right at the beginning of the table from the moment that research is designed. The philosopher or bioethicist can function as a benevolent gadfly to ensure that concepts employed, be it genes or autism or development, are straightforward and consistently used by researchers in interdisciplinary projects. I will point out the many issues at stake in research projects and how these reinforce outdated and dualistic views on life that are not conducive to a progressive science. An ethical research practice is a self-reflective practice. I contend, perhaps too quickly, that in the case of genes, this means adopting a long-term, developmental, and dynamic perspective on life.

In the second part of the book, *Chance and Creativity*, I continue on the path of a developmental outlook on life. I argue that such an outlook implies that bioethics focuses less on what we can control, for example, what we can know from our genes and more on dealing with chance and uncertainties. I use ideas from Alfred North Whitehead and process philosophy to challenge a representational approach to bioethics. I describe concepts from Stuart Kauffman and others to introduce aspects of creativity in life and explain how they view life as fundamentally creative. I also describe new materialist entanglements of ethics, ontology, and epistemology to argue that, given this creativity of life and the universe, ethics is implied all the way down. Moreover, describing

     https://doi.org/10.11647/OBP.0320.02

organisms and practices, and choosing how to describe them, is not a mere representation but creates possibilities for our world's future. Living is finding creative solutions and reflecting on the worlds we want our practices to create. Each 'chance encounter' entails possibilities. Our choices and words are deeply ethical. The fact that we make our worlds depending on the things and creatures we encounter, and hence also make ourselves, means that understanding life is understanding experience.

In the third part of the book, *Experience*, I return to one of the central tenets of bioethics, that of bio*medical* ethics. I describe how there is a rich literature on concepts of disease in the philosophy of medicine— understanding what we mean by health and disease influences how we think about the ethics of medicine. Given my commitment to development and process philosophy, I shall describe a thoroughly biological and normative way of looking at pathology and health, that of Georges Canguilhem. I shall conclude that if we take the normativity of concepts such as pathology seriously, we should pay attention to experiences and situated knowledge. Such sensitivity to experiences is relevant in the encounter between an individual patient and their caregiver and in evaluating the impact of systemic decisions. Ensuring an ethical scientific and clinical practice entails including the viewpoints and explicitly paying attention to those who have held marginalized positions in healthcare. If we want to understand what health and pathology mean for different people, this means engaging honestly with those who have been ignored.

Acknowledging the situatedness of general, clinical, and scientific knowledge, in particular, means that bioethical practice must be intersectional. In the fourth part, *Troubles*, I develop ideas around intersectional and speculative bioethics. I use Donna Haraway's notion of *Staying with the Trouble* to argue that bioethics should not strive for quick fixes or easy answers to complex questions. It means caring for such a future and thinking with philosophers, scientists, and everyone whose interests are at stake. In a ruined world, the private and the political are intrinsically intertwined. In times of existential principles and moral theories are helpful tools that can help us approach specific problems, but they do not provide straight answers. Our focus must be on a liveable future for everyone, both human and other-than-human.

How to get to such a future is not so much a puzzle to be solved as it is an exercise in creativity and playfulness. At the same time, staying with the trouble also means thinking of ourselves as trouble and the troubles we make. It means being aware of the world-making of humans and other beings. In the fifth part, I will use the concepts of risk, autism research, animal ethics and my own journey in a computer game as examples of practical ethical questions and methodologies that urge us to stay with the trouble of our own and the world's limits.

This book is not the result of the solipsistic endeavour of one academic philosopher. Its title, *Chance Encounters*, is as much a reference to those instrumental in forming the ideas in this book as it is to a specific view on life and creativity. It is thus dedicated to all friends and colleagues who have become friends that have shaped my thinking. 'Chance' (or 'sjans') in Dutch is colloquial for 'good luck'. I am fortunate to collaborate with a brilliant team of inspiring people. Dear team and dear colleagues, you know who you are. This book is yours as much as it is mine.

PART ONE: SCIENCE

In which I describe the deep entanglement
of ethics and science.

The sciences of the Anthropocene are too much contained within restrictive systems theories and within evolutionary theories called the Modern Synthesis, which for all their extraordinary importance have proven unable to think well about sympoiesis, symbiosis, symbiogenesis, development, webbed ecologies, and microbes. That's a lot of trouble for adequate evolutionary theory.

– Donna Haraway (Haraway, 2016, p. 49)

I don't see anything out there that is not nature. Everything is nature. The cosmos is nature. Everything I can think of is nature.

– Ailton Krenak (Krenak, 2020, p. 7)

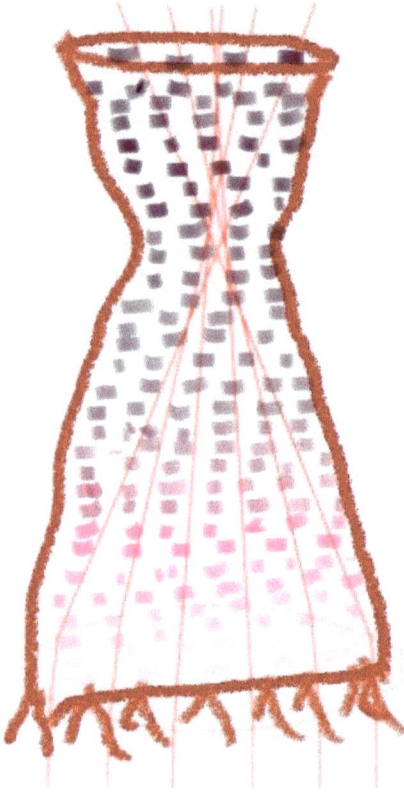

Microbial seasonal colours in a cooling tower of Tihange nuclear power station.

How to express the relationalities of the micro-organisms within a cooling tower of an electric power plant and its milieu.

From: Research on attunement with microbes in cooling towers and lungs.

Sketch by Bartaku, 2022[1]

---

1   This sketch is part of a new cross-disciplinary Bartaku Art_Research strand featuring the internal and external entanglements of cooling tower microbiomes. It was made during The Institute for Relocation of Biodiversity research residency at wpZimmer, workspace for performing arts, Antwerp, 2022, https://wpzimmer.be/nl/residencies/diversifying-and-locating-relocation/

In this Part, I aim to describe the deep entanglement of science and ethics and what this means for bioethics. I do this not from 'science and values' studies or a poststructural perspective but, firstly, to reimagine the position of bioethics vis-à-vis science and suggest that bioethics can be an endeavour in the spirit of Van Rensselaer Potter. This means that the bioethicist's role starts at the inception of a research project. Secondly, I use the topic of genes as an example of how certain ideas about biology have shaped how we think about ethics. The topic of genes also allows me to introduce my ontological commitments to developmental ('epigenetic') perspectives on organisms.

3. Research Ethics all the Way Down

The Curious Case of Paulo Macchiarini

A biochemist and oncologist, Van Rensselaer Potter did not consider science and ethics separate endeavours. In his 1971 book *Bioethics, A Bridge to the Future,* he argued that bioethics should be a bridge between science and humanities to allow for a genuinely ethical science and ethics that aim to make such a science possible (Rensselaer Potter, 1971). In his view, bioethics is not merely biomedical ethics, focused on issues of consent and risks, but it is the foundation on which good science is built. Since then, many ethicists and scientists have thought this viewpoint was somewhat simplistic: science and ethics remain separate disciplines with different goals and methodologies. Bioethicists are welcomed in biomedical research projects, for example, to think about proper consent procedures and, if the project team is open to it, to engage stakeholders and query the opinions of patients and the general public. The idea that ethicists and philosophers could contribute to solidifying the conceptual framework on which a research project is built is not yet widely accepted. True enough, philosophers of science have done precisely this work, but their conceptual work is not often seen in the light of its ethical relevance. In what follows, I will argue that bioethicists, philosophers of science, and scientists can and should work closely together. I will use the example of genes and concepts of genes to illustrate why thinking about conceptual foundations is of utmost importance for bioethicists and why they should join forces with philosophers of science and demand a place at the project table of biomedical and scientific projects.

 https://doi.org/10.11647/OBP.0320.03

One of the biggest scandals in research ethics is the case of the Italian thorax surgeon Paulo Macchiarini (De Block, Delaere and Hens, 2022). He claimed to have devised how stem cell populated donor trachea, and even artificial trachea could be transplanted into living persons. He performed these procedures on several patients with damaged trachea. Seven of the eight patients who received artificial transplants died due to the process, leading to Macchiarini being indicted for aggravated assault in the autumn of 2020. Discussions about the case have focussed on how charismatic con man Macchiarini had fooled prestigious journals, funders, and renowned universities alike. For example, there was much media attention for how he conned NBC television producer Benita Alexander into thinking they would be married in Italy, blessed by the pope. Macchiarini was outed by several whistle-blowers and by the relentless work of Belgian thorax surgeon Pierre Delaere, who wrote several letters to the journals that published Macchiarini's research and the ethics committee at the Karolinska Institute in Sweden, where Macchiarini was employed.

Nevertheless, it would be wrong to merely see the Macchiarini case as an exceptional case of mythomania and conmanship. Granted, the degree of the fraud and the tragic consequences are far-reaching and shocking. At the same time, there likely must have been something in the mindset of all the Macchiarini supporters, very often scientists, that would have enabled the scandal to occur. Moreover, the same attitude has led to enthusiasm in specific fashionable and promising areas of medicine, such as stem cell research and genetics in general. However, it has also led to underfunding in more mundane areas of science, such as research into infectious diseases. This enthusiasm for fringe science is understandable: we want to believe in the progress of science and scientists' ability to do great things. People tempering the enthusiasm are considered killjoys or even Luddites.

Professor Pierre Delaere, a thorax surgeon, might be seen as one of these killjoys when he argued for the impossibility of Macchiarini's procedure in 2015. He claimed that, given the nature of the trachea, not a mere standalone pipe but an intricate structure populated with veins, the technique Macchiarini had invented was logically impossible. It could only lead to suffering and death. He got the following reply from the ethics committee:

> We find that the issues raised by Professor Delaere are of a philosophy-of-science kind rather than of a research-ethical kind. Accordingly, the Ethics Council concludes that, on the backdrop of the examined issues, Professor Delaere's allegations of scientific misconduct are unfounded.

This reply is telling but, at the same time, not surprising. It sheds light on the presumed tasks of ethicists and research ethics committees. Their job is, so suggests this quote, to assess aspects of research that include proper informed consent, risk assessment, and return of results policies. These aspects were indeed also suboptimal in the Macchiarini case. However, there seems to be an assumption that it is not the task of the ethicists or the ethics committee to query the conceptual underpinnings of the science itself. The quote suggests that *philosophers of science* may have something to say about these underpinnings. However, the specific task of these philosophers of science in the process of ethics approval is unspecified. It seems that science should be left to handle its conceptual affairs.

We may wonder whose task it is, however. In fundamental research, hypotheses may be confirmed or rejected through new research. Usually, not much harm is done to human beings while doing fundamental science, although the practical applications of such science may do great harm. Nevertheless, the question remains whether there is a moral duty to ensure that research is at least plausible, given the scarce resources available to fund research projects. For example, consider the Human Brain Project, a ten-year research project funded by the European Commission. This project aimed to simulate human brain functioning in a computer to understand better the origin of conditions such as Alzheimer's disease. However, two years in, the project's goals and underlying assumptions were questioned, and Henry Markram, the project leader, was forced to step away from it (Frégnac and Laurent, 2014). Projects such as these are often presented as risky science—science with a high likelihood of failure—but at the same time, with immense potential. Therefore, money should be set aside for such fringe science. Otherwise, we may miss out on great opportunities. However, there is a fine line between a risky but promising science and a fluke. After all, when Italian neurosurgeon Sergio Canavero announced that he wanted to perform a first 'head transplant', this was called 'fake news' and unethical by bioethicist Arthur Caplan (Caplan,

2017). Nobody in their right mind would fund research into head transplants. However, both the head transplants and the Human Brain Project are based on the same flawed assumptions. These assumptions suggest that who we are, our cognition and our identity are primarily based on our brains. It is assumed that the rest of our body is a tool we can easily replace with someone else's body or a computer. Moreover, in the case of the Human Brain Project, the additional assumption is that how our brain functions can be simulated on a computer. These philosophical assumptions have been investigated by philosophers of mind and philosophers of biology who have critically examined the existing scientific and philosophical arguments. The feasibility or even adequacy of a brain-in-a-computer simulation is built on shaky grounds: it is very probable that humans, and organisms with brains in general, are not (solely) their brains but their entire bodies. It is also likely that cognition does not work 'like a computer'. Perhaps artificial intelligence, even so-called 'strong' artificial intelligence, is possible if we agree on what is meant by the concept of intelligence itself. However, such strong intelligence will not be analogous to human brains and will not be attained by mimicking brain functions. Hence, projects such as the Human Brain Project should have been rejected for funding precisely because of arguments from the philosophy of science.

The same holds for experimental clinical procedures such as the ones performed by Paulo Macchiarini. Pierre Delaere's objections were indeed of a 'philosophy of science' nature: he argued that the operations performed were, in principle, doomed to fail. As we deal with a clinical practice involving patient procedures, the ethical implications are immediately evident. A risk assessment by an ethics committee should not only weigh the harms and benefits of a technique. It is true that, were such a procedure to work, it could help many people. However, as Delaere's arguments demonstrated, the Macchiarini case is not analogous to the first heart transplants, where the risks were worth taking because the procedure can, in principle, work. There is no potential benefit in artificial trachea transplants as there is no chance that they will work. However, in prestigious research projects such as the Human Brain Project, where the dangers are not directly affecting actual patients, there is an ethical imperative to build them on conceptually sound grounds. Conceptual reflection in medicine has been done by philosophers of medicine and clinicians practising philosophy of medicine, such as Edmund D. Pellegrino, Jeffrey P. Bishop and H. Tristram Engelhardt, *Journal of Medicine and Philosophy* and the book series *Philosophy and Medicine*. I will return to some of the concepts from philosophy of medicine in chapter 11. What has become clear from the Macchiarini case is that conceptual work is relevant for research ethics as well and may even save lives.

When writing this book, the COVID-19 pandemic is still in full force. It is a wake-up call to scientists and bioethicists alike that an infectious disease caused by a virus can have devastating worldwide consequences. Of course, there are many countries where viral and other epidemics have always been present. We may wonder if Western hubris has caused research funders, researchers, and bioethics to be primarily interested in technologies and science such as stem cells, genetics, and computational models of brains. We can only speculate what the world would look like if more research had been done about the mechanism of infectious diseases or coronaviruses. Therefore, I contend that one of the tasks of ethicists who think about the ethics of scientific practices is to dare to question the underlying assumptions of that science. Hence, I argue that the philosophy of science and bioethics should inform each other to improve the science they reflect on.

What Is Philosophy For?

In the previous paragraphs, I argued that if we want to assess the ethics of a specific research protocol, it is not enough to take the science itself for granted and focus on research integrity questions and research aims. Instead, thinking about conceptual matters is also an ethical endeavour. In pandemic times, in the light of fake news, conspiracy theories and vaccine hesitancy, all hampering the progress in beating the virus, we often hear that 'science knows best' and must fight ignorance. Although I, in principle, agree with this statement, it does not mean that scientists never make mistakes or that concepts and assumptions in scientific projects are clear or sound. Later in this first part, I will use the examples of nature and nurture and of genes and environment to demonstrate how seemingly straightforward concepts are no longer so when we look at them with further scrutiny.

I argue that part of the task of bioethics involves thinking about concepts and presumptions made in biological and biomedical sciences, a job that traditionally befell philosophers of science. Still, we may wonder whether philosophy is really up to that task. Indeed, philosophers can investigate what kind of arguments scientists use and even their outlook on reality. However, can philosophers evaluate scientific concepts? Maybe the idea that a philosopher must have a place at the table with scientists from the conception of a research protocol is an example of hubris. Philosophers must not pretend that they know everything about the nitty-gritty details of the techniques used in technical detail. Their place must be at the margins, and they should be grateful even to have been allowed a place at the project table. Nevertheless, I think the reluctance to have philosophers and other humanities scholars involved from the conception of a project onward is unfounded. It is precisely because a philosopher or, in my case, an ethicist may not be fluent in the vernacular that they are also valuable at this stage. They can query inconsistencies and ask for clarifications. They can function as benevolent gadflies in science projects. They do not take concepts or presuppositions for granted and ask annoying conceptual questions like the primordial gadfly Socrates did in Greek society. Philosophers should, at the same time, cooperate with science in good faith, with benevolence, and as colleagues with scientists as they have the same goal. The relation between philosophers and ethicists, on the one hand, and exact scientists, on the other hand, is one of mutualism rather than parasitism. Moreover, philosophers can identify different forms of knowledge necessary to understand a phenomenon in all its aspects. In Part Three, I will argue that an ethical science of life automatically implies investigating experiences and different modes of thinking. Philosophy, and more broadly, the humanities, can add this as a valuable component to a research project.

The reader may object to the philosophy and ethics I refer to here. Indeed, philosophy is more than the philosophy of science, and philosophers have other jobs to do than help make scientific research projects better. It is true that for many, philosophy seems to be a grand endeavour, trying to think through humankind's relationship with nature, with God, and what makes us unique. Preferably this endeavour is undertaken with the help of the grand philosophers that came before us. This type of philosophy may still be worth doing, even considering humanity's significant existential challenges. Nevertheless, I think the philosopher we need, and most desperately need in desperate times, works from the trenches of research practices. In this respect, the idea of philosophical plumbing, conceived by Mary Midgley, is helpful (Midgley, 1992). Midgley is perhaps best known to the general public for taking issue with Richard Dawkins' idea of the selfish gene (Dawkins, 2016). For her, the idea of the selfish gene was conceptually unsound, and I think nowadays we can agree with her, as my further elaboration on the concept of the gene will show. However, she was attacked as 'not knowing the science' by proponents of the selfish gene. How much more productive and beneficial could it have been, for genetic science in general, to have a Mary Midgley at the table querying basic assumptions and helping make science better? In an earlier book, *The Myths We Live By*, Midgley argues against scientism (Midgley, 2004). The idea of a value-free science is naïve: science has its myths and beliefs it takes for granted, although they are not 'scientific' per se. An example is the myth of geniuses accumulating knowledge, discoveries, and inventions.

Midgley compares philosophy, metaphorically, to plumbing. Like the pipes in plumbing, philosophy consists of hidden structures that we need that support us but that we do not think about very much. Moreover, plumbing engages with the messiness, and even crap, of the world. Midgley argues against sterile principles and lifeboat examples, in which ethics is reduced to a deliberation on the fair distribution of scarce resources. Philosophers should acknowledge and engage with actual situations and irreconcilable facts. 'Complexity', she states, 'is not a scandal'. Philosophers, just like plumbers, should get their boots dirty. Plumbers also deal with water and the unruly and unpredictable effects of water. They create flow when things get stuck. Philosophers deal with life and all its discontents. Plumbers work on joints and bring disjointed things back together. Philosophers, according to Midgley, are especially useful at the intersection of different disciplines. Philosophers, like plumbers, look at the bigger picture of the system. They can point out how everything is connected. Midgley writes:

But of course, philosophy is the key case, because it is the study whose peculiar business it is to concentrate on the gaps between all the others, and to understand the relations between them. Conceptual schemes as such are philosophy's concern, and these schemes do constantly go wrong. Conceptual confusion is deadly, and a great deal of it afflicts our everyday life. It needs to be seen to, and if the professional philosophers do not look at it, there is no one else whose role it is to be called on (Midgley, 1992).

In her last book, *What Is Philosophy For*, Midgley argues that philosophy is more than ever needed as an ally to science in desperate times (Midgley, 2018). It is required because, like the plumber, philosophy can shed light on hidden structures, connections, and specific places where these connections go wrong. She ends the book by stating,

We shall need to think about how to best think about these new and difficult topics — how to imagine them, how to visualise them, how to fit them into a convincing world-picture. And if we don't do that for ourselves, it's hard to see who will be able to do it for us (Midgley, 2018, p. 208).

If we conceive bioethics as applied philosophy of life, I think the comparison of the plumber is adequate. In what follows, I shall give one example where there is a certain amount of philosophical and scientific plumbing. Still, more is needed, using the concept of nature and genes and their normative implications. Furthermore, although most individual scientists will acknowledge the shortcomings of a mechanistic view of life, it remains the case that conceptual schemes such as the dichotomy between genetics and environment still play an unarticulated role below the surface. For example, they play a role in what counts as objective science and in which scientific projects are considered worthy of funding. The nature-nurture discussion has also been a recurrent theme in bioethics, albeit sometimes not overtly acknowledged: think about specific discussions on cloning or embryo editing. It seems that we bioethicists should not only do the plumbing as contractual work for other disciplines but also fix our own sinks.

4. Against Dualisms

When I was writing this chapter, in the autumn of 2021, the discussion about whether children should be vaccinated against COVID-19 was in full force. A growing number of people argue that the risks of a COVID-19 infection are relatively low for children. Therefore, they should not receive vaccines only recently developed, as some consider these experimental vaccines. I will not go into detail about the ethics of COVID-19 vaccination here. Children are not a homogenous group, and there are groups of children at a higher risk for having adverse effects of a COVID-19 infection. Some of these children will not receive the vaccine for medical reasons. I think preventing the spread of the disease is an act of solidarity with those with underlying health issues. There is a tendency amongst some people to minimize COVID-19 by stating that 'only the weak and the old' run risks. These are ageist and ableist assumptions that do not sit well with me at all. We could argue that children are somehow exempt from a duty to solidarity, and we should not expect them to undergo the same risks as adults for the sake of others. That may very well be the case, but at the same time, children are gradually educated into solidarity. Moreover, it is in everyone's best interest that the pandemic is over as quickly as possible. Since much of the spread is now happening at schools, vaccination of children seems sensible. Still, at this point in the book, I do not want to present an in-depth argument favouring the immunisation of children. I want to focus on one argument against the vaccination of children that tells of a specific conceptual scheme that underlies our thoughts, both in bioethics and science. An idea often found in lay people's discussion on vaccination is that being infected with the actual virus and attaining 'natural' immunity is better than the artificial immunity that vaccines would induce. Especially in children, who often are not very sick from COVID-19, this would be the preferred route to take.

  https://doi.org/10.11647/OBP.0320.04

What strikes me here is the idea of 'natural' and 'better'. People seem to intuit that manufactured or artificial vaccination does something unnatural to our immune system and that this is not the preferred route to achieve immunity. In the case of COVID-19, a new virus our system has never met, this argument based on nature seems strange and maybe even unwarranted. We could make other distinctions. For example, we could say it is better to 'train' our immune system with a controlled vaccine rather than an active and new virus. However, this is not the automatic conclusion that people draw, and this is testimony to how certain dichotomies profoundly influence our thinking and the normative conclusions we draw. Understanding these conceptual schemes underlying our reasoning and, if necessary, confronting them is intrinsic to the ethics of life. In what follows, I shall give the example of two such dichotomies intimately related: nature versus nurture and genes versus environment. I will point out that they have normative implications and that we should be aware of where they come from and how they influence our thinking. Biological science and bioethics that is forward-looking will, in my view, transcend such dichotomies.

Debating Nature and Nurture

In their 2001 book, *Design for a Life. How Biology and Psychology Shape Human Behavior*, Patrick Bateson and Paul Martin wrote:

> The best that can be said of the nature/nurture split is that it provides a framework for uncovering a few of the genetic and environmental ingredients which generate differences between people. At worst, it satisfies a demand for simplicity in ways that are fundamentally misleading. (Bateson and Martin, 2001, p. 138)

They demonstrate that genes and environment do not simply add up together. Instead, they compare development to cooking: merely emphasizing the individual ingredients does not make sense when cooking a meal. It is the process of combining and merging everything that matters. Nevertheless, despite scientists' acknowledgement of the importance of environmental factors, 'nurture', and regardless of the practical difficulties of studying the environment, the discussion between nature and nature is ongoing. In 2019 and 2020, there was upheaval on social media about whether studying the relation between 'race' and IQ was a valid research question. To set the record straight from the beginning, I do not consider this the case. As I will argue further down the line, I think one explanation for the persistence of the nature and nurture dichotomy is that it carries normative weight. The IQ and race discussion struck me as an example of how despite all the nuances scientists exhibit about genes and environment. The nature-nurture dichotomy seems deeply ingrained into how we think about living beings' traits and behaviours. We consider what is part of someone's 'nature' as static and resistant to change unless we deploy invasive methods like gene therapy. What we have acquired through our lifetime, through 'nurture' and interaction with the environment, seems intuitively more readily changeable.

Take the example of IQ. Some have argued that your genes and ancestry primarily determine your IQ. Choose your mate wisely if you want a child with a high IQ. For others, IQ is primarily malleable by education. If you wish to raise your child's IQ, you can stimulate their intelligence through education, brain training, etc. So, the outcome of the question 'is it nature or nurture' has normative implications. If our goal is to 'increase IQ', the way forward will be different if we believe it has a genetic basis or if we think it is primarily influenced by education. Our most profound convictions on whether certain traits are mostly nature or nurture may affect what kind of science we should do, thus influencing outcomes. Think about the example of autism. The idea that autism is an innate, lifelong characteristic of a human being leads to the fact that much autism research has focused on finding (presumably causative) genes. The fact that researchers have found genes that run in autistic families then serves to prove that the original assumption is correct.

In what follows, I will argue that the question 'is it nature or nurture' is often not a good way to approach specific questions regarding the explanation of traits or development. We should, in my honest opinion, stop asking ourselves this question. Again, I acknowledge that most present-day scientists hold the same view and consider this discussion obsolete. However, despite the more nuanced vision that many scientists have, the nature/nurture question keeps popping up in the scientific accounts of popular media. Why is that so? Why does whether a specific trait is due to our 'nature' or our 'nurture' seem so important? Why do we want to situate something either in genes or the environment? Why do we consider genes and environment as different spheres but spheres with equivalent explanatory power? Of course, others have asked themselves this question as well. Timothy D. Johnston asks himself precisely this in a paper in 1987 called *The persistence of dichotomies in the study of behavioural development*. In the abstract, we can read:

> The inadequacies of dichotomous views of behavioral development that oppose learned and innate behavior, or genetic and environmental determinants of behavior, have long been recognized. However, they continue to exert a powerful influence on current thinking about development, often by way of metaphors that simply recast these old ideas in a more modern technical vocabulary. (Johnston, 1987).

It is 2021, and we are still asking ourselves that question. In autumn 2019, I was asked to give a webinar on this topic for the Belgian VCOK (Vormingscentrum Opvoeding en Kinderopvang) and Steunpunt Adoptie. Indeed, many adopted persons, adoptive parents, and donor-conceived offspring have questions about the relative weight of genes versus education. I warned them that my talk would be philosophical and that I would not provide an answer. I told them that I considered every possible reply to this question nonsensical. This is an example of how it can be better to 'stay with the trouble' as a bioethicist. At the same time, studying its history to understand a phenomenon, such as the nature-nurture dichotomy, is an excellent way to start. It allows us to see the messiness and complexity of what, at first sight, seem clear-cut concepts. In what follows, I shall describe the history of the discussion, starting from the 19th century. I acknowledge that asking whether something is 'inborn' or acquired may be as old as humanity. Francis Galton, a cousin of Charles Darwin, received the credit for coining the terms nature and nurture in 1874. He wrote *English Men of Science: Their Nature and Nurture*, in which he noticed that intelligent people, in that period presumably smart men, were often related to other intelligent men (Galton, 1895). This caused him to think that intelligence was something familial. So, he decided to use the terms nature and nurture, which he thought sounded nice, as is apparent from the following quote:

The phrase 'nature and nurture' is a convenient jingle of words, for it separates under two distinct heads the innumerable elements of which personality is composed. Nature is all that a man brings with himself into the world; nurture is every influence without that affects him after his birth (Galton, 1895).

Indeed, today, when we think about nature, we often still think it refers to an essence, to what is innate. When we think about nurture, this is what is influenced by education and the environment.

Nevertheless, the nature-nurture discussion is related to other discussions that may be centuries old. For example, there is a philosophical discussion between *preformation* and *epigenesis*, which is connected to how the *form* of an organism takes shape. People who believe in preformation think that the form of organisms is present from the outset and merely *unfolds* when they develop. Some have argued that the belief in genes as a blueprint for organisms, as was often championed in the second half of the last century, is essentially preformationist. If we believe what we will become is defined in our genes, this is present from our conception and resistant to many influences. The term *epigenesis* is reminiscent of the more recent epigenetics but is not synonymous. I will come back to their relationship later in this chapter.

Epigenesis assumes that an organism's form is not wholly predetermined from the start but is shaped by other influences. Such influences can come from inside an organism: for example, the location of a cell in the body influences the function it performs. However, these influences could also come from outside, from physical and psychosocial factors (Maienschein, 2000). There is also the aspect of *time*. Are an organism's characteristics fixed from conception, or does it acquire them over time? There is the aspect of *place*: is what an organism becomes encapsulated within it, or is it under external factors? What are these external factors, then? Do we inherit characteristics from our biological progenitors, or do we acquire them throughout our lifetime? Are genes the cause of our behaviour and traits, or do environmental influences primarily cause these? All these nuances are part of the nature-nurture debate, and scientists have investigated different aspects.

For example, let us examine the distinction between innate versus acquired ('learned') behaviours. In the first half of the twentieth century, behavioural biologist Konrad Lorenz reflected on the concept of 'instinct', which is innate (Richards, 1974). He investigated the songs of birds. Do birds still sing a particular song when deprived of their parents' example right after birth? If they do, the behaviour (singing a specific song) is innate, instinctive. The birds have evolved to exhibit the behaviour regardless of whether their parents teach it. However, another scientist, Daniel Lehrman, disagreed with this. He took on a developmental ('epigenetic', as in 'epigenesis') perspective (Lehrman, 1953). He argued that even these deprivation experiments, where you remove newborn animals from their mothers, do not prove that something is innate or acquired. Development does not start when an organism is born. It begins when an organism is conceived. Some would argue it starts even before that, as I discuss when I talk about epigenesis. There is consensus that the prenatal environment is highly influential, as vindicated by recent findings in epigenetics, and I shall discuss this later. Organisms learn before they are born. We hear the songs that our mother sings for us in the womb. Moreover, as epigenetics findings demonstrate, a pregnant woman's experiences also influence gene expression in the foetus. With that, we have come to the discussion on genes. When pondering the causes of traits or behaviours, the question is often: Is it in our genes or caused by the environment?

Before we look at these complex interactions and relations, I would like to delve into other explanations of why we want to situate the causes of conditions or behaviours in genes or the environment, and especially in genes. How we think about genes and how we consider whether something is attributable to nature and when something is attributable to nurture has a consequence on how we feel about a specific condition or trait. However, if we look at people's behaviour merely due to their nature or their genes, we risk not taking them seriously as human beings. We risk seeing them simply as mechanisms and reducing them to their 'biology'. For example, we may decide that intelligence is fixed. It would mean that it is pointless to stimulate children to increase their intelligence. Instead, we might think they should be sent to the right school that caters to their maximum attainable level of intelligence. This is a scary thought, not in the least because it abstracts from the hopes and dreams of the children in question.

Genes-Environment

In the twentieth century, the nature-nurture distinction became almost synonymous with gene-environment. Stating that something is attributable either to genes or the environment or even to an interaction between the two seems to have similar normative implications as saying something is attributable to nature or nurture. Nevertheless, the idea that genes and environment are two distinct spheres of influence conveys something even more potent. By presenting genes and environment as juxtaposed, genes have some special status: their explanatory power is on the same level as the environment. Moreover, encapsulated within an organism, genes strengthen the idea of a hard border between that organism and the environment. Whether this is an accurate description of how organisms function is under debate. The persistence of the importance of genes is related to findings and successes in medical genetics, as I will argue later. However, the automatic link that people often make between health and genes may also be problematic. Medical science has a primary therapeutic aim. When researching disorders and diseases and their causes, we do not merely want to understand how they came about but to which extent this knowledge can help us progress therapeutically. Hunting for genes may not be the best way to go about it. Also, bioethics' love of genes over the last few decades may have to be curbed. Suppose it is, as I firmly believe, also the task of the bioethicist to question the goals of specific research projects. In that case, it is imperative to examine the impact of focussing too much on the promises of projects in genetics and the like. First, let us investigate some concepts, histories and possible misunderstandings concerning genetics in the following paragraphs. Philosophers of science may be well acquainted with what I describe in the following sections and may want to skip it.

For many, 'nature' has become synonymous with 'genetic' and 'nurture' to the various environmental factors influencing development. The distinction between genotype (our genetic makeup) and phenotype (the organism with all its traits) was framed by Wilhelm Johannsen (1857–1927) in the early twentieth century (Johannsen, 1911). Suppose we present it in such a way as two distinct types. In that case, it appears to be a simple calculation: genotype plus the environment is a phenotype, and phenotype minus environment is the genotype. At the time of Johannsen, DNA structure was still unknown, but people already used the term 'gene' to refer to a unit of inheritance. Thomas Morgan's discovery that there were actually 'genes' on chromosomes (1866–1945) solidified the idea that genes are essential for inheritance (Morgan, 1910). This solidification eventually led to the modern synthesis of evolution and Mendelian genetics, as a mechanism was discovered ('genes') by which inheritance and evolution would work.

Furthermore, when Franklin, Watson, and Crick discovered DNA structure ('the double helix'), we could finally see the molecular structure of genes. This discovery reads as a straightforward story of scientific progress, and partly it is. However, discovering the molecule is insufficient to explain genes' almost mythical significance in many societies today. The rise of information science probably exacerbated this idea. At around the same time as discovering the double helix, there was a rise in research into cybernetics in the mid-twentieth century. The idea of codes and written programmes that can be read and executed has probably helped enshrine the idea of a genetic programme and organisms built up from a genetic blueprint. We now think of genes as things we can read and from which we can predict certain traits or diseases. This fact is probably equally attributable to molecular genetics and information sciences maturing together as disciplines than to mere scientific progress alone. The 20th-century view of genes as the primary difference-maker for traits and behaviours has become popularized in books such as *The Selfish Gene* by Richard Dawkins (Dawkins, 2016). For developmental systems theorists, genes do not have special status: they are one cause among many others. I will return to the importance of the concept of development later on. Others take a more intermediary position. For example, Kenneth F. Schaffner does attribute some special status to genes in his book *Behaving: What's Genetic, What's Not, and Why Should We Care?* (Schaffner, 2016). Genes, he argues, are a bit special, as they provide a linear explanation and are 'necessary condition explainers' (Schaffner, 2016). Moreover, they provide powerful tools to investigate behaviour. Still, Schaffner argues, we need to consider them in the complex pathways and networks in which they function, so he does not subscribe to the gene-centric view of the mid-twentieth century (ibid.). I will not take a stance in the debate here but confess that I am sympathetic to trying to steer attention away from purely genetic explanations. That is not to deny that genes are exciting and relevant or that we should stop investigating them. However, we may miss meaningful opportunities to consider organisms differently by focusing on genes.

When I talk about genes, I may give the impression that a gene is a pretty straightforward concept. However, genes can have different meanings. We have already described the 'gene' as the unit of inheritance, as we can deduce from Mendel's research. A gene then denotes which characteristics in the organism's phenotype are inherited from its progenitors. Besides that, Franklin, Watson and Crick have also discovered that 'gene' corresponds to a molecular structure. Specifically, the gene is part of the DNA that codes for a protein. However, that does not mean that the first meaning of the gene, the gene as the unit of inheritance, which we can deduct from looking at characteristics and biological parents, overlaps one on one with a piece of DNA code. The reality is far more complex.

Population genetics, specifically behavioural genetics, has influenced ideas about genes and how these are presented in the media. A good example is the reporting on a gene 'for bullying'. In 2019, at least in Belgian media, it was stated that 'genes influence bullying behaviour'. Let us look at the bullying study itself, claiming that bullying would be mostly 'genetic' (Veldkamp *et al.*, 2019). If we read such findings in the media, we may intuitively assume that bullying is unavoidable for those people with specific genetic variants. We may think that a bullying child does not control their behaviour and that it will be hard to change their behaviour. We may assume that they are probably part of a very annoying family. However, the scientific findings come from population genetics, meaning they convey something about population variance, not individuals. Although population genetics may describe general tendencies that may, to some extent, be relevant for individuals, this relevance is far more implicit than is often assumed. David S. Moore explains this very well in his book *The Dependent Gene. The Fallacy of Nature versus Nurture* (Moore, 2003). I have based the explanation in the following paragraph on this book. For population genetic studies, researchers often look at monozygous twins to determine how much of the variance in the population can be explained by 'heritability' and how much by 'environment'. Researchers denote the component of behaviour that the environment cannot explain with heritability. This 'heritability' is then a number between zero and one, so 'schizophrenia is 0.49 heritable' would translate to: 'in a given population, we can explain 49% of the individual differences regarding schizophrenia through genes' (ibid.). Moore describes a gruesome thought experiment. It is based on what Mark Twain once said about teenagers and deals with the heritability of intelligence. Imagine, Twain said, you put four boys who are not family of one another in four barrels. You give them the same food. The environment remains 100% the same. If you measure the boys' intelligence, you could point out that these are due to genes. In this population of teenagers in a barrel, intelligence differences are 100% due to 'genes'. Imagine that four genetically identical children- monozygotic quadruplets or four clones- are raised in a different environment (Moore, 2003). You raise one child on the international space station, one in a family of wealthy industrials, one with a group of native people from Brazil in the rain forest, and the fourth in China's countryside. If you now measure their intelligence, you could say that all differences are due to the environment because they have the same genes. The heritability will be low. This finding does not say much about whether intelligence is more genetic or environmental, although it conveys something about their relationship. It also does not say much about how the intelligence of a specific individual came about. In behaviour genetics, scientists are talking here about variance in a particular population level, not about the relative percentages of genes or environment that have contributed to the phenotypes of specific people.

Nevertheless, how people communicate such studies often suggests that genes and environment are separable realms, even when discussing individual people. Population geneticists acknowledge that genes and environment are not separable realms—typically, when explaining variances in a population, it is not as simple as 'genes' (G) or 'environment' (E). They investigate the third factor of the interaction between genes and environment (G x E). There are genes that code for the interaction with the environment. Even if we factor in G x E, these percentages do not reveal much about individual organisms' development. If behavioural geneticists say that a trait or behaviour is, for example, 25% environment, 25 genes and 50% their interaction, they are not explaining the cause of the trait or behaviour. Instead, they are saying something about the variance in a population. The traits and behaviours cannot causally be divided into genes or environments. If a study reports that 'bullying is 70% genetic', this does not mean an individual bully is 70% deterministically defined by their genes to bully. It also does not mean that there is, on the molecular level, a 'gene for' bullying. Population genetics is a statistical science, and it is very technical. This complexity may explain why popular media often translate these findings into simple 'gene for' language.

However, it is also true that genes seem to have a special status in science and popular imagination. Looking for a genetic explanation or even a genetic 'cause' for a particular trait or behaviour seems to have a specific appeal. I was struck by how much money and time has been spent finding 'the gene' for autism. There has been little reflection on why it would be so important to find the gene for autism rather than understanding what may help autistic people in their daily lives. I think that this desire to find an ultimate cause is understandable. Dennis Noble has described it accurately in his book *The Music of Life* (Noble, 2006). He states that 'complexity is uncomfortable'. It is only human to look for simple explanations for complex phenomena. If we try to explain a complicated thing such as behaviour, it is comforting to assume that we could find at least one part of the explanation in the genes. I also think that there is an additional explanation. I have discussed different meanings of 'gene': they are a piece of the DNA molecule that codes for a protein or explanation for statistical variance. At the same time, genes have also become a powerful cultural icon. At least in Western culture, we think genes are essential to our identity. When it comes to identity, they have explanatory power. In their book, *The DNA Mystique*, Dorothee Nelkin and Susan Lindee state that in cultures where many people no longer believe in a god, biology—especially genes—may have taken that role (Nelkin and Lindee, 2004).

> Introductory biology is presented as a valid, truth-seeking endeavor, untainted by religious, political, or philosophical commitments. It places human beings in a meaningful universe, providing ways of understanding relationships between ethnic and racial groups and between identity and the body. Biology, in a very real sense, has become a philosophical and religious domain, and the genome itself has become a guide to the human condition. (Ibid.)

Genes give us a handhold, a fixed identity. Think about the saying 'it is in my genes'. This cultural idea of the gene is critical to take with us if we think about how we think about genes and the ethical implications.

We may naively think that scientific researchers try to answer whether a trait is nature or nurture do so without a preference either way. However, researchers work in a specific context from a particular conviction. Let us go back to Francis Galton, who observed that many intelligent people have family members who are also smart, which would prove that intelligence is heritable and innate (Galton, 1895). Galton is primarily known for his eugenic thoughts. Of course, we can easily take the step from 'if something is in your nature, you cannot change anything about it, and then the right thing to do is marry the right person'. In the Soviet Union, people thought about these issues differently. In the spirit of communism, such ideas were inconceivable: people could be educated, but their genes did not determine them (Dugatkin and Trut, 2017). Everything was in their genes. One of the best-known Soviet scientists, although some would not call him a scientist, was Trofim Lysenko (1898–1976). His thoughts exemplified 'environmentalism', not in the sense of advocating for the environment, but in thinking that everything is nurture, and we can only attribute a few characteristics to 'nature'. This type of thinking fits into the communist ideology, which led to a setback for genetic science in the Soviet Union. It may have been responsible for the collapse of the agro-system, which caused massive famine and millions of deaths (Borinskaya, Ermolaev and Kolchinsky, 2019; Fresco, 2021). The disdain for these 'environmentalists' is apparent from the quote cited in *Design for a Life* by Bateson and Martin. They quote a cynic stating that 'environmentalists seem to believe that if cats gave birth in a stove, the result would be biscuits' (Bateson and Martin, 2001, p. 12). I was not able to trace whose quote this was.

Moreover, based on the previous discussion, we could conclude that right-wing politics is more associated with a gene-centric view, ancestry and eugenics. A left-wing and progressive view is more readily associated with the environment, malleability, and social mobility. However, Maurizio Meloni succinctly explains in his book *Political Biology* that this link is not straightforward: 'environmental approaches in principle lend themselves to normalization and enhancement endeavours, and an appreciation of genetics can sometimes lead to an appreciation of diversity' (Meloni, 2016). I shall come back to this when discussing epigenetic determinism. Nevertheless, both gene-centric thinkers and environmentalists consider nature and nurture or gene and environment as two separate spheres, each having independent explanatory power. However, questioning gene centrism does not mean attributing everything to the environment, nor does it imply that some traits may be more flexible than others.

Of course, how we think about genes is influenced by and influences science, specifically biomedical science. The fact that genes have acquired such importance is also related to the fact that there has been substantial progress in medical genetics regarding the correlation of specific diseases with certain mutations in genes. In *Between Nature and Nurture*, Evelyn Fox Keller describes how medical genetics, in the same way as medicine in general, is a comparative science: you take a baseline of a 'normal' (non-pathological) individual and you compare it with a diseased individual, and you look for a significant 'difference maker' (Keller, 2010). Mutations in genes or chromosomal abnormalities correlate with the development of certain diseases such as Huntington's disease, Mucoviscidosis and Neurofibromatosis and are the difference makers. Finding such difference makers has led to the idea that we may also see a genetic cause for other diseases, even for general behaviours and traits. In this spirit, several projects were ongoing at the turn of the century. Think about the Human Genome Project, in which the entire genome was unravelled. Another example is HapMap, a project in which people have tried to find the genetic basis of certain diseases. We are twenty years later, and the results of these projects are sobering in that they have mainly demonstrated the complexity of the genome rather than finding direct causal links between genotype and phenotype.

Moreover, Evelyn Fox Keller states in *Between Nature and Nurture* that several problematic steps are taken in 'gene for' language in medical genetics. She states that:

> its language invites us to lose sight of the complex moves—first, attributing the cause of a phenotypic difference to a genetic mutation; second, assuming that the presence of a mutation automatically signals the presence of a gene; and third, attributing responsibility for the trait in question to the gene in which the mutation is assumed to have occurred— that are routinely made in effecting this shift from comparative to individual. (Keller, 2010, p. 47)

Keller describes how medical geneticists rely on molecular sequences to find mutations or alternative sequences that are thought to be responsible for specific traits. Such mutations do not always correspond to a protein-coding gene. Hence, talking about a 'gene for' may be misleading. It is not because we find a molecular difference in the DNA that correlates with disease status that this automatically means that this stretch of DNA also corresponds to a gene. You may wonder why it is relevant that we make this distinction. Whatever is on the DNA is 'genetic', and if we think about the importance of genes, we may very well think about anything in the DNA molecule. However, the question remains why something with various meanings in science has acquired such mythical status with almost limitless explanatory power. Perhaps the idea of the gene feeds into our desire for simple explanations.

Furthermore, the idea that a gene causes disease or that a stretch of DNA is responsible for a trait is valuable information. It can explain a particular feature or disorder straightforwardly. Here comes the next big jump in medical genetics and medicine. There is a heartfelt belief amongst medical professionals and patients alike that if we can only find the cause of a specific disorder, this will bring us a long way towards fixing or 'curing' the condition. This belief is problematic. First, let us assume that the claim that specific mutations in DNA, be it in protein-coding genes or non-coding parts of DNA, actually 'cause' diseases, disorders or traits. It does not automatically imply that this *specific* finding will easily translate into clinically valuable practices. Although pharmacogenomics and gene therapy have been much hyped, the possibility of fixing aberrations in the DNA is unlikely to happen soon. As I will argue later, it is probably also a priori impossible in many cases. When I interviewed clinical geneticists a couple of years ago about the value of finding a genetic explanation for autism, they remained very vague regarding the therapeutic value of such findings (Hens, Peeters and Dierickx, 2016b, 2016a). In some instances, for example, if autism is associated with specific syndromes such as Fragile-X, this knowledge can contribute to the clinical care of the particular child. Some geneticists pointed out that we may correlate genetic findings with responses to certain drugs in the future. They also point out the psychological importance of finding a biological 'cause' of autism: this would, in some cases, relieve parents from guilt, which may be therapeutic. Many of these so-called benefits remain speculative.

The most often quoted benefit of finding a genetic explanation autism professionals gave me was giving parents of an autistic child reproductive options. Suppose a child's autism was correlated with a genetic mutation that parents could pass on to future children. In that case, they could make reproductive decisions: either decide not to have children or use reproductive technologies such as preimplantation genetic testing (embryo selection) to avoid having a child with that mutation. I shall not detail the ethics of reproductive decisions per se. We have time to do that when I discuss risks in Part Five. I want to point out that this aim is far from our ordinary conception of a therapeutic purpose. It is uncertain how this would help with these children's challenges. I do not want to downplay the importance of genetic findings from a scientific point of view: correlating mutations in DNA with certain traits or disorders is a critical step in understanding the development of organisms. Doing so with the expectation that it will have immediate therapeutic benefits may be misguided.

We need more than a simple correlation between aberrant sequence and phenotype if we are interested in therapeutic medicine. Indeed, I come to the second point that Keller raises. She states:

> As to the possibility of other kinds of treatment or prevention in a particular individual carrying the aberrant sequence, this depends on understanding something about the biological function that has been disrupted by the identified change in sequence. Such a quest takes us beyond the analysis of phenotypic differences induced by mutant forms. Indeed, it requires an altogether different kind of analysis, almost always one of a far more difficult nature. (Keller, 2010, p. 48)

Keller stresses that DNA is embedded in an immensely complex and entangled system of interacting resources. Understanding this system requires an altogether different analysis and probably a different type of (medical) science. To know how traits or disorders develop, we must not merely understand what difference a gene makes in medicine but the causal pathways. If the goal is to truly understand the causes and development of disorders and even behavioural atypicalities such as autism, we need to study the development over time. This study implies understanding DNA, genes, and their interaction with other factors.

Today, confronted with such criticisms, scientists and philosophers alike will often deny that they still think a strict ontological distinction between nature and nurture is relevant. The geneticists I talked to over the last decade acknowledge that most diseases or behavioural phenomena are not the results of one or several genes alone. Some have told me that the reductionist view on genes that I and others seem to question dates back 40 years and is obsolete. I grant that in individual talks with researchers, their opinion is far more dynamic and nuanced. It is a truism that genes interact with their environment. Still, 'gene for' language is prevalent in a large number of publications; the 'gene for' autism quest is a case in point. Although all these publications admit that there is more to the story than mere genes, far less research is done into what this 'more than' actually means. Also, over the past years, I have spent my fair share of time at conferences for genetic or autism research. I have seen many cases in which researchers have claimed to have made an autistic mouse or an autistic fruit fly using gene technology. It demonstrates that mechanistic and even reductionist views on genetics and behaviour still govern research practice, although individual researchers may know better. Indeed, a vast proportion of research money goes to genetic research. That there may be a clash between researchers' views on organisms and the actual research they practice should give us pause. One of the reasons, I think, why there is so much focus on genes is that genes are circumscribed things. We can hunt for them. Using all the new technologies available for molecular analysis, researchers can apply for a four-year doctoral grant to find a correlation between a genetic variant and a trait. The environment, however, is everything else that is not a gene. How can we ever tackle that? What is needed for that is advanced systems biology tools and powerful AI. Then we may dream of factoring in the vast unknown that is the environment. Then science will know it all and truly understand how certain traits or diseases come into existence. At least concerning autism, the topic I have worked on for the last six years, this seems to be the prevailing story. Billions of euros/dollars/pounds have funded the search for a genetic basis of autism over the last decades. This sort of made sense, as autism seems to run in families, which implies genetics. Hunting for a gene in a specific population is feasible in the four years of a typical research project. Many papers that result from these endeavours acknowledge that the genes, if found, are not the final answer: they are often so-called risk factors or susceptibility genes. The authors of these papers state that part of the explanation is in 'the environment'. Investigating these environmental factors is the subject of further research, which will often not happen, given how scientific practice is organised. Indeed, I think there are relatively few examples of research programmes that investigate such complex entanglements of different factors, regardless of the promises of precision medicine and AI, because development is highly complex to analyse. Such research seems to be impossible to integrate into current research funding schemes.

Nevertheless, I also believe that what we can gain by studying the development of disease rather than its primary cause is valuable. Medical genetics has shown that most diseases and traits result from the interaction between genes and their environment. We do not merely have to 'read' genes or find relevant genes to understand such complex interactions. Instead, we need approaches from systems biology and complex models to consider the impact of the environment throughout an organism's development. The hunt for a specific gene for a particular condition or treatment is perhaps somewhat obsolete. However, I must also stress this does not mean that genes would not play a role or would not be necessary anymore. They are part of an organism's functioning, and in that respect, studying them can help understand the intricate system that a cell or an organism is.

Epigenetics[1]

When discussing the meaning of genes and the artificiality of the nature-nurture discussion, authors often name recent findings in *epigenetics*. I also admit I am guilty of using 'epigenetics' in this way, like a magic wand that can prove reductionists and determinists wrong. I first learned about epigenetics while doing my PhD between 2007 and 2010. In this PhD, I investigated ethical issues regarding using DNA samples from

---

1   For those who want to delve deeper into the science of epigenetics, microbiome, development and symbiosis, I recommend the intriguing and accessible *Ecological Developmental Biology: The Environmental Regulation of Development, Health, and Evolution* by Scott F. Gilbert and David Epel (Gilbert, 2015).

minors for genetic research. The paediatric angle allowed me to explore common assumptions concerning informed consent, risks, benefits, and return of research results. At that point, I did not question the belief that we can learn much from our genes and that, to some extent, we can use genes to predict traits and disorders. However, I read *Evolution in Four Dimensions* by Eva Jablonka and Marion J. Lamb (Jablonka and Lamb, 2014). A seed of doubt was sown: maybe the bioethicist's focus on genes is not all that warranted. What does this alternative vision of evolution and development mean for bioethics? During those years and my first years as a postdoc, epigenetic findings found their way into news outlets. We have known for a long time that what a pregnant mother eats or inhales may affect the development of the foetus.

Molecular findings in epigenetics, enabled by new techniques that allowed for the investigation of methylation patterns throughout the genome, have laid bare the molecular link between the environment and the nucleus. The environment has become concrete in its effects on the cell. If we talk about epigenetics now, we think about these molecular effects first and foremost. As such, 'epigenetics' is an integral part of the science of genetics; the next step after discovering the double helix in the mid-twentieth century and discovering techniques to read what is written in the DNA, from Sanger sequencing to microarray analysis to whole-genome sequencing. We can now go further and find out what controls gene expression. We can investigate what makes a skin cell a skin cell and what makes certain genetic risk factors associated with a disease phenotype in specific individuals and not others.

I discuss my ideas with both geneticists and bioethicists alike. Geneticists tell me I apply a mythical status to epigenetics while it is a mundane subject for them. Bioethicists also wonder why epigenetics would change how we discuss ethical issues concerning new technologies. Indeed, some ethical questions, such as the fact that epigenetics may contain identifying information or the fact that what pregnant mothers do or eat affects the offspring's future health, are somewhat analogous to the discussions we had on the ethics of genetics. Still, epigenetics can point us to something beyond, a different way of thinking about life. Such an entangled and processual view of life is not new. Nevertheless, the emphasis on the mechanics of genetics in the wake of the modern synthesis has somewhat obscured this view.

Before deciding whether epigenetics can change how we look at organisms and change a bioethicist's way of thinking, it is good to reflect on its different meanings. These various meanings have something in common: the importance of development, and a developmental perspective. I have already mentioned the word epigenesis, a concept sometimes claimed to be unrelated to epigenetics as a molecular science. Epigenesis is a theory on the development of organisms as formulated by the German physician and naturalist C. F. Wolff in contrast to preformation (Wessel, 2009). A preformationist view assumes that an organism's eventual form is already there from conception onwards. Think about the 17th-century idea of the homunculus. After discovering gametes, some researchers at that time assumed that either the sperm cell or the ovum would contain a 'little man', which would merely become enlarged during development. If we consider that the combination of genes received when sperm and ovum fuse is the thing that determines what an organism will become, this idea is somewhat preformationist. Therefore, some people have suggested that neo-Darwinians have preformationist tendencies. However, even the most fervent neo-Darwinist would acknowledge that our experiences and environment play an essential role in what we will ultimately become. After all, Darwin himself stressed the importance of encounters with changing environments as a motor for evolutionary change in species. Undoubtedly, the same must be valid for the development of an individual organism. I shall argue further down the line that certain preformationist tendencies have some guiding role in bioethics and are closely linked to concepts of identity.

In the mid-twentieth century, Conrad Waddington introduced the idea of the epigenetic landscape (Creighton and Waddington, 1958). Waddington used the image of the landscape with valleys and hills to describe the development of a phenotype. Every cell has the same nuclear DNA, but they develop into specific types of cells depending on the place in the organism. Waddington describes two crucial concepts. Plasticity is the ability of a given genotype to give rise to different types of cells in response to environmental circumstances, such as the place in the organism (Creighton and Waddington, 1958). Canalization is the adjustment of the developmental pathways to bring about a uniform developmental result despite genetic and environmental variations

(Creighton and Waddington, 1958). Imagine a little ball running through a landscape of branching valleys: it is the cell that starts as a generic kind of cell and then, depending on the environmental circumstances, is sent through a specific canal or valley, ending up as a specific type of cell. Some cells follow the canal or valley of a liver cell if they are in the right part of the body, and other cells will become skin cells or blood cells. Imagine also that the landscape is rearranged a bit. For Waddington, it is not the genes that influence the landscape but the network of genes. The network or the landscape can change because there are changes in many genes. A minor rearrangement will not significantly affect the cells' trajectories because of the canalization. However, if the landscape is completely rearranged, this will severely impact development. It is important to note that canalization and plasticity are not opposite. They imply each other. Canalized development requires some plasticity to adapt to different circumstances. Furthermore, adapting to different circumstances means being fixed enough to withstand total annihilation. Indeed, stability requires dynamics to keep systems stable (Jablonka and Lamb, 2014; Jablonka, 2016).

Waddington described the epigenetic landscape as networks of genes controlling development. Nowadays, epigenetics refers to molecular mechanisms that may or may not be inherited. If you were, like me, educated in the last decades of the 20th century, among the things you may remember from your biology classes was the idea that characteristics that an organism acquires during its lifetime are not passed on to offspring. This idea has been enshrined in collective memory by referencing the views attributed to Jean-Baptiste Lamarck. A seminal image to illustrate Lamarck's misguided ideas is that of the giraffe, acquiring 'by use' a longer neck to reach the tree's higher-up leaves. Darwinism, so our biology teachers would say, corrected this idea: it was not so that giraffes extended their necks during their lifetimes. On the contrary: giraffes born with longer necks, and thus able to reach the higher leaves, were more likely to survive until reproductive age and produce offspring with longer necks. Biology teachers also quickly pointed out how these characteristics were passed on. They were versed in what is known as the modern synthesis of biology. Darwin's ideas were revolutionary but lacked a mechanism. Through the appreciation of Mendel's laws, mid-twentieth-century scientists proved the necessary mechanism by laying bare the structure of our DNA in the double helix. Richard Dawkins's seminal work, *The Selfish Gene*, further enshrined this idea of genes as replicators (Dawkins, 2016).

Genes thus conceived are remarkably indifferent to the organisms they are located in. The genes provide the blueprint from which the organisms are built. In line with twentieth-century enthusiasm for cybernetics and information science, people imagined genes as a *code* composed of a nucleotide system of four letters. This picture represents what has become known as the central dogma of genetics. The central dogma dictates that DNA is transcribed into RNA and translated into proteins. The idea is that the arrows between DNA to RNA to proteins are unidirectional: there is no feedback from proteins to RNA to DNA. This central dogma remains unchallenged: the DNA molecule does not change after conception, with some rare exceptions such as mutations. Moreover, it is the same in different cell types.

However, what is remarkable is not the inertness of the DNA molecules but that genes have acquired such a predominant status in how we view life, including bioethics. Genes have slightly different meanings depending on the scientific discipline that deploys the term. For example, the gene explains variance in a population in behaviour genetics. In molecular genetics, the gene is a meaningful piece of our DNA. Let us now take a generalised meaning of 'gene' as a starting point: a gene is a piece of DNA that meaningfully transcribes and *translates* into protein. In this meaning, the gene is also inert, we are born with a specific genetic makeup, and exceptional cases, such as bone marrow transplants or nuclear incidents aside, we will die with it. This fact is in itself trivial, and I will not challenge it. What is not trivial is how the gene has acquired such predominant status in the way we think about the nature of human beings. 'It is in our nature' or 'it is in our biology' has become almost synonymous with 'it is in our genes'. Indeed, organisms experience many environmental influences, but the baseline code from which everything starts is the genes. This idea has thoroughly influenced bioethics, as I shall argue later.

The central dogma cannot explain the development of an organism. This fact has been known for quite some time. A 21st-century biology teacher would probably nuance the above picture of the gene's predominance, versed as they may be in recent findings concerning gene expression. They may point out that although each cell has the same nuclear DNA, cells belong to different cell types, more than 200 in the human body, to be specific. Cells of different types perform other functions: a liver cell performs differently than a skin cell. So, some mechanisms must explain how different genes are expressed. The environment of the cell in the body must somehow inform this mechanism. They may also point out that although monozygotic twins share the same DNA, they are different. Throughout their life, they may be susceptible to other diseases. They develop distinct personalities. In the same way, in a more science-fiction-like example, we can imagine a dictator desiring a human clone as a progeny to continue his reign. Although the likelihood that this clone will share similar tendencies to their father may be higher than in the case of an individual sired more traditionally, the clone's developmental trajectory and the actual history will differ. They will not be mere duplicates. Indeed, as I will elaborate further, biology also has a history.

The 21st-century biology teacher could then elaborate on the mechanisms that enable such context-sensitive on-and-off switching of genes. Although many of these mechanisms are still not entirely known, a few have been studied to some extent. For example, there is DNA methylation. Methylation occurs at the level 'on top' of the DNA: Methyl groups, tiny carbon compounds compared to DNA, can be added or removed from specific regions. As a result, genes that are 'underneath' these groups become accessible or inaccessible for transcription. If a methyl group blocks a particular gene, this gene cannot be transcribed. The gene becomes accessible and transcribed again if a methyl group is removed. These methylation patterns can nowadays be checked by 'Genome-Wide Methylation Analysis'. Another mechanism is histone modification. Imagine DNA as wrapped around a specific protein, histone. If DNA is wrapped more tightly by the histone, specific genes, some regions of the DNA become less accessible for transcription. If DNA Is wrapped more loosely around the histone, the transcription factors can more readily access the gene. Histone modification seems to be more flexible and transient than DNA methylation. Certain types of RNA, such as microRNA (miRNA), are also implied in gene expression.

What is already interesting here is that these epigenetic changes happen under the influence of an external stimulus and can happen under the control of DNA. They may also depend on the milieu they inhabit within the organism and potentially be susceptible to the input of the environment in which the organism is. Such environmental influence can be the physical environment. Think about the influence of particulate matter on methylation. These factors could be psychological or even social, such as stress. It seems as if the more we know about this molecular link between DNA and the environment, the more organisms are intrinsically linked with their milieu. That genes and the environment interact is straightforward, but the actual specifics of these interactions become apparent in the study of epigenetics. Indeed, although the concept of 'gene' may mean different things in different scientific disciplines, as I have described before, at least there was some consensus on what constitutes a gene. However, giving environmental molecular effects a central stage in how we think about biology also opens up the vision of human nature. Human nature is no longer what is fixed, what we have from birth, but becomes adaptive throughout one's life. Why would what is written in our genes have precedence over what we experience in our environment? This dynamic and open aspect of the nature of organisms is one of the central themes of this book, and I shall return to it later.

Right now, let us go back to our discussion of evolution. Indeed, our 21st-century biology teachers will probably tell a more nuanced story about evolution than their 20th-century counterparts. Epigenetics has become known among the general public as the mechanism that challenges the idea that organisms do not pass on acquired characteristics to their offspring. Although the specific mechanisms seem not well understood, many studies have now demonstrated that acquired characteristics can be passed on from generation to generation. For example, in an article from 2017 in Science, Adam Klosin and colleagues describe how environmental factors influence gene expression and how these changes can be passed on to the next generations (Klosin *et al.*, 2017). The fact that environmental factors influence gene expression is in itself not spectacular. Klosin et al. 2017describe an experiment where C. Elegans worms were genetically modified to emit light when put in a warmer environment. If the researchers put them at approximately 20 degrees Celsius, the worms would glow only slightly. If the researchers raised the temperature, the gene that caused fluorescence was turned on, and the worms started to glow more intensely. However, the worms retained their intense glow when the temperature was lowered again. Moreover, their progeny inherited the glow and even seven generations further down the line, glowing worms were born. If five generations of C. Elegans worms were kept warm, this characteristic was passed on to fourteen generations.

There are also examples of transgenerational effects in other animals, including humans. A seminal example is that of women who had early pregnancies during the Dutch Hunger Winter in 1944–1945 and had children who were more prone to obesity. It is suggested that this effect also occurred in the grandchildren (Painter *et al.*, 2008). If we want evidence for germ-line epigenetic modification, we could focus on whether the father's experiences may be transmitted to grandchildren. It has been suggested that some sensory experiences can be passed on to the next generation based on experiments with rodents. For example, in a study, male mice were exposed to a particular smell and then received a shock. The researchers mated these mice with unexposed females. Their offspring were also comparatively anxious when confronted with the smell, and even the grandchildren of the frightened male mice were wary of the particular smell (Dias and Ressler, 2014). It is hypothesised that this is due to epigenetic inheritance. That such inheritance could occur is a mystery. Scientists have assumed that any epigenetic markers that would originate from a father's experience would be wiped clean from sperm cells and hence have no effect on the development of the offspring. The inheritance of acquired characteristics is against our intuitions. People look for different explanations. For example, the actual epigenetic markers may not have been inherited. However, the environment in which the behaviour occurs may be replicated, and this replication is perhaps under genetic control. There have been suggestions that what looks like the true inheritance of molecular changes is the inheritance of a specific niche or environment. The phenotype may be rebuilt in each generation rather than inherited. Indeed, whether there can genuinely be an inheritance of acquired characteristics is still contended by some authors. Studying the inheritance of epigenetic changes in organisms such as worms is hard to neglect. Admittedly, C. Elegans is an entirely different type of animal from vertebrate animals such as human beings. Whether acquired characteristics could be inherited in the latter type of animal remains to be demonstrated. For some scientists, it is unthinkable that epigenetic markers such as methylation patterns could be transferred through germ cells. They believe there would be a complete erasure of epigenetic markers upon conception. Others disagree.

In any case, an oocyte is an entire cell with a cytoplasm, not just nuclear DNA. The metabolic conditions in the fertilized oocyte are influenced by lifestyle and environment. Thus, they could play a role in transgenerational imprint and influence epigenetic programming during embryogenesis. As such, this mechanism could allow for a kind of Lamarckian inheritance.[2] The epigenome mirrors our metabolism and the ncRNA spectrum. The entanglement between the mitochondrial metabolism, ncRNAs and DNA methylation constitutes the epigenome: Even if all DNA methylation is wiped, the metabolites and the ncRNA form a kind of backup to reconstruct the DNA methylation patterns. In this sense, epigenetics/epigenomics is the interaction rather than the methyl patterns themselves. What happens in the cytoplasm is equally relevant to what happens in the nucleus. In this light, epigenetic inheritance is perhaps intelligible. At the same time, we do not need to accept this genuinely Lamarckian type of inheritance to acknowledge the intergenerational effects of epigenetics and their consequences on health and personal responsibility. For example, certain studies have suggested that maternal smoking increases the child's risk of asthma and the likelihood of a grandchild developing asthma (Bråbäck *et al.*, 2018). This influence happens regardless of whether the child (the 'second generation') smokes. We do not need inheritance 'through the germline' to account for this: the foetus in the smoking woman's uterus already had oocytes (egg cells). The grandmother's smoking can directly influence these.

Genes are the things we are born with that do not change, and we inherit them from our biological progenitors. They seem to have an equal standing next to the environment: genes and environment are equally valid factors influencing one another. In the previous paragraphs, I

---

2   I would like to thank Wim Vanden Berghe for explaining this to me. Readers who like to read up on the controversy may consult the following papers: Daxinger and Whitelaw, 2010; Skinner, 2014; Whitelaw, 2015; Guerrero-Bosagna, 2016; Houri-Zeevi et al., 2021; Robles-Matos et al., 2021.

have argued for a more predominant place of 'the environment' in how we think about life. Life is, in this way, not merely synonymous with organisms built up from genes. We know that gene expression is under environmental control. However, what the environment is has remained vague. It can mean the cellular environment. The things we eat. Or could it be the city we live in or the parenting styles we were subjected to? The stress we experienced, or even our parents experienced? The latter is suggested by a study on the epigenetic transmission of PTSD during the genocide in Rwanda (Perroud *et al.*, 2014). Studying the mechanisms in the cell implies we must be more specific about the concept of the environment. Maybe the coarse distinction between physical, psychological, and social environment is no longer sustainable. Still, the idea that 'everything is biology' will feel too reductionist. Perhaps the physical, psychological and sociocultural should no longer be considered separate spheres but as different aspects of a more comprehensive biological realm that is dynamic and teeming with meaning.

5. Development and Ethics

Development and Environment

In the previous chapter, we have seen how epigenetics is a term with different connotations. It bears a family resemblance to the much older term *epigenesis*, which denotes a way of looking at how organisms acquire a specific form. Adherents of the theory of *epigenesis* believe that an organism develops its form during development in interaction with the environment. Preformationists, on the contrary, believe that the form of an organism is already defined from its conception. The environment can either be the milieu inside or outside of an organism. The more recent term epigenetics refers to contemporary research in molecular biology that studies the intracellular mechanisms of gene expressions. These mechanisms can be controlled by genes or the environment and work throughout an organism's lifetime. I have also discussed the concept of the epigenetic landscape as Conrad Waddington devised it. He described a network of genes that we could consider a landscape which guides the development of a particular cell towards a specific endpoint (Creighton and Waddington, 1958). Important concepts here were *canalization* (the mechanism that causes the development of a cell to take a specific path, a particular 'valley' in the landscape) and *plasticity*, which introduces the possibility of adapting to changes.

The different meanings of epigenetics have at least two aspects in common. First, there is the idea of *development*. The emphasis is on how organisms develop and interact throughout a lifetime. They 'lay down a path in walking', to quote the late cognitive scientist and enactivist

 https://doi.org/10.11647/OBP.0320.05

thinker Francisco Varela (Varela, Rosch and Thompson, 1992).[1] Development is not confined to what happens in the womb or the first phases of an organism's development but continues from conception to death. Secondly, there is an emphasis on the environment. Epigenetic changes occur under environmental control. We have seen that whether something is 'caused' by genes or environmental factors stresses a false dichotomy. It suggests that these are two well-defined spheres on equal footing when explaining the causality of traits, behaviours, and pathologies. We have seen that the concept of 'gene' is far from straightforward. Even more complex is the idea of the environment. The environment can denote behavioural factors, such as lifestyle and nutrition, and factors in the physical environment, such as pollution. There can be psychological factors such as stress and trauma. Moreover, our culture could also be considered a factor contributing to gene expression. And besides cultural influences on gene expression, we can also look at culture itself in terms of development and epigenetics.

Quite a few scholars have theorised the relationship between genes and culture. Think about the seminal work by Richerson and Boyd, *Not by Genes Alone* (Richerson and Boyd, 2006), in which they describe how culture changes the nature of human evolution and, at the same time, how human beings change a culture. Hence, culture and human biology evolve together. Iddo Tavory, Eva Jablonka, and Simona Ginsburg elaborate on cultural epigenetics (Tavory, Jablonka and Ginsburg, 2014; Jablonka, 2016). They build on Waddington's epigenetic landscape. They write about how a cultural system is a dynamic entity into which individuals are introduced, in which they develop, and to which they contribute. Groups of individuals become socialized into a culture. Culture can be considered a social landscape comparable to Waddington's original 'epigenetic landscape' compiled from genes. Each social community is a niche construction with particular dynamics and life patterns that evolve and develop. The inhabitants maintain these customs and practices over time for these customs to become canalized. Each community has its own culture. Concurrently, these smaller communities are part of bigger social landscapes, so more complex regulatory structures are required to help maintain or canalize each of them.

---

1   Varela was inspired by the poem *Traveler, There Is No Path* by the Spanish writer Antonio Machado.

Tavory, Jablonka and Ginsburg illustrate this using two examples. First, there is the example of the Orthodox Jewish society in LA's Beverly-LaBrea neighbourhood. This culture is thriving amid a transgressive, secular youth culture. Several factors help to maintain the religious tradition. There are well-established geographical limits: community members attend the same places and schools. Every person has multiple obligations in the community, and people do not have much time for anything else. They wear particular clothes and thus distinguish themselves from others outside their community. In this way, the specific tradition has become canalized. To a large extent, the culture is resilient against external pressures. Tavory and colleagues also give another example: urban poverty in the USA (Tavory, Jablonka and Ginsburg, 2014). They describe a cycle of poverty: people born into urban poverty tend to be poor themselves, and it is tough to break this cycle. We can ask ourselves why this is the case. There seem to be many social-cultural factors that lead to this situation. They include the structure of the state and the schooling system, and to some extent, biological and epigenetic factors such as alcohol and drug consumption. Moreover, when someone succeeds in escaping this vicious circle of poverty, they usually disappear from this society, leaving no positive influence. There is also a geographical factor. A poor neighbourhood has certain geographical boundaries, and there may be attractors such as cheap housing or the availability of drugs that make it hard to break through these boundaries. The cycle of poverty is canalized.

These two examples suggest that a cultural epigenetic approach offers little hope of improving suboptimal situations, such as urban poverty. Epigenetics does not automatically lead to less deterministic conceptions than a purely genetic view of the world. However, the Waddingtonian network approach to culture and biology describes how certain traits and behaviours have become canalized dynamically. The ideas of canalization and plasticity leave an opening for change. Indeed, Waddingtonian networks are not set in stone. They can change and reshuffle. Understanding canalization and plasticity can help us intervene and reshuffle the valleys into desirable paths. In what follows, I shall return to the challenges and opportunities of epigenetics for ethics.

Development and Ethics

What is so special about the ethics of epigenetics that differentiates it from the ethics of genetics? We have already discussed that epigenetic changes can be transgenerational, maybe even heritable. This extended timeframe poses some extra challenges when we think about responsibility. We can assume that pregnant mothers have some responsibility for the unborn child. Many would consider a pregnant woman engaging in binge drinking irresponsible if she knows the dangers to the future child's health. However, if epigenetic findings suggest an influence by the behaviour of men long before they even consider siring children, how should we, for example, evaluate the responsibility of teenage boys who smoke if we know that this may affect the health of potential future children? Surely, fifteen-year-old boys should preferably not smoke for their health, but it would be strange to claim they are responsible for future children they might never have (Hens, 02/2017). Another relevant aspect when discussing the ethics of epigenetics is that epigenetic markers may be more readily reversible than genetics. It may be easier to wipe out or induce a methyl mark than alter a gene (Nakamura *et al.*, 2021). This reversibility offers many opportunities for therapy, but it also raises some interesting ethical questions. The idea of precision medicine suggests a shift towards more preventive rather than curative medicine and entrenches the idea of taking responsibility for one's health. However, if epigenetic markers can more readily be changed, this may suggest a move back to more curative medicine. Consider the scenario of the smoking fifteen-year-old boys. We should perhaps not bother telling them to stop smoking, as we will be able to wipe out the deleterious influence this has on their future offspring. Undoubtedly, the fact that something can be cured does not relieve us of the responsibility of preventing harm from happening in the first place. The same goes for systemic responsibilities such as pollution. The idea that we may eradicate the nefarious epigenetic effects of pollution in the future is comforting. However, it feels wrong to allow harm to occur because we can fix the consequences later. At the same time, we cannot count on the fact that this biomedical knowledge will ever be available. Perhaps the most important new aspect that epigenetics brings is that of unpredictability. Epigenetics is about interaction with the milieu. It positions organisms as fundamentally open to their environment. We must factor in an amount of chance. I shall discuss chance, indeterminacy and creativity more in Part Two. For now, suffice it to say that keeping in mind both the reversibility and indeterminacy of epigenetics can function as a shield against deterministic interpretations of epigenetics and eugenic interpretations.

Authors have warned that epigenetics, and focusing on the environment, does not automatically imply more plasticity and malleability. The idea that we are defined not only by our circumstances and lifestyle but also by the experiences of our ancestors may suggest that we are determined by more than merely our genes. Indeed, epigenetics determinism, being determined by both genes and environment, may even be worse than genetic determinism. It suggests that there is no relief from the traumas of our grandparents or great-grandparents. Contrarily, the idea that the epigenetic layer is malleable also opens the way to what Eric Juengst and colleagues have called 'epi-eugenics' (Juengst *et al.*, 2014). If the aim is to create better people, the idea that we can tinker with environments and their molecular effects opens up more possibilities. *Developmental Origins of Health and Disease* (DOHaD) research stresses the importance of environmental influences at the earliest points in life, at conception and in utero. It thus raises questions about the responsibilities or even duties of pregnant people towards the health of their offspring. Popular media has already translated specific findings regarding a mother's duties, for example, the claim that eating bacon and eggs during pregnancy will make your child smarter. In their *book Blinded by Science*, David Wastell and Susan White point out the consequences of neuroscientific and epigenetic research (Wastell and White, 2017). They describe the possible implications of focusing on the first three years of development. Parents may feel pressure to do everything right and make no mistakes when it comes to parenting their young children. Stressing this 'window of opportunity', in which children's brains are flexible, has spawned a whole industry of tools, toys and techniques to 'improve' your child. In Part Three, I shall question the idea of improvement itself. For now, I believe that these presumptions make the same mistake: they assume, just as people did before about genetics, that epigenetic knowledge will lead to more control over who we are and who we can become. A developmental approach, with epigenetics as one of its molecular proofs, may ultimately show that the desire for control is misguided. As I shall argue in Part Two, we need a kind of ethics that engages with unpredictability, chance, and lack of control.

I shall not go into more detail regarding the ethics and consequences of epigenetics. Bioethicists, sociologists, and lawyers have already written about this extensively. For an overview of the discussion from the last decades, the reader can consult the excellent literature review by Charles Dupras, Katie Michelle Saulnier and Yann Joly (Dupras, Saulnier and Joly, 2019). Instead, I shall give one example of how a more developmental view of organisms can shed new light on the assumptions we have taken for granted, specifically reproductive ethics.

Certain concepts of development are thoroughly influencing how we approach bioethical issues. This influence becomes apparent when we think about specific discussions in reproductive ethics. A common assumption is that at least our (numerical) identity is fixed at conception. This assumption is linked to the conception of personhood in certain religions: think about the Catholic church and its absolute prohibition of abortion. They argue that personhood starts at conception. Conception is defined as the merging of genes from the sperm and the ovum. When considering reproductive ethics, the idea that identity is created at the point of conception carries much normative weight in secular bioethics too. This idea is related to the relevance that the (non-)identity problem seems to have for reproductive ethics. Derek Parfit has described the non-identity problem in his seminal book *Reasons and Persons* (Parfit, 1984). He asks us to imagine a fourteen-year-old girl who wants to become pregnant. We would probably advise her to wait until she is older and/or has more stability in life. Postponing would give the hypothetical child a better chance in life. However, Parfit asks us to consider for whom this would be better. It may be better for the girl herself to focus on her studies first before engaging in the demands of parenthood. But we cannot say that it would be better for 'the child', as the child she conceives in her late twenties will be a different child than the one she might give birth to if she became pregnant now. After all, in theory, a different sperm and ovum will produce a different child in the future. So, leaving aside the potential harm to the girl herself, can we say that the child that would be conceived now is harmed?

Moreover, the environment may be very different for the girl and the child 10 or 15 years in the future, making predictions about well-being nearly impossible. The background to this thought experiment is whether harms are always personal, affecting a specific someone, or whether situations themselves can also be harmful, even if it is difficult to pinpoint precisely for whom it is harmful. This example is classified as a non-identity problem and has had a significant impact on authors' discussions in papers on both reproductive and environmental ethics (Del Savio, Loi and Stupka, 2015). For example, William P. Kabasenche and Michael K. Skinner describe the potential transgenerational harm of the pesticide DDT (dichlorodiphenyltrichloroethane). The use of DDT as a pesticide has been banned for decades. However, recently it has been used to control malaria in some regions of Africa. Its use is linked to the transgenerational inheritance of kidney, testis and ovary disease. Hence, the use of DDT to protect the current generation's health will affect future generations' health. This idea raises an ethical dilemma, which is made even more complex if we factor in the non-identity problem. Presumably, using DDT to prevent malaria will affect who is conceived at what time. If we stop using DDT, the future generation will be different from those born if we use it. This creates a paradox. The very people we are trying to save in the future will potentially never exist in the first place. To whom do we have a responsibility, then? M. C. Roy, Charles Dupras and Vardit Ravitsky have discussed the implications of the non-identity problem to reproductive technologies (Roy, Dupras and Ravitsky, 2017). The non-identity problem is relevant if the technologies affect which child will be born, not if we affect a child or embryo already in existence. Hence, epigenetic harms that occur before conception, through manipulation before fertilization, will affect identity (and bump up against the non-identity problem). However, epigenetic harms or influences, such as the culture medium, that affect the embryo *in vitro* will not be identity affecting, as the embryo will be the same.

In what follows, I shall investigate how a developmental view of life can challenge the importance we attribute to numerical ('genetic') identity. It is by no means my intention to solve the non-identity problem, just to demonstrate how different ways of looking at identity can shed a different light on decades-old discussions. In 2020, two months before

the COVID-19 crisis broke out, I was at a workshop near beautiful Lake
Geneva hosted by the Brocher Foundation. It would be my last 'IRL'
conference for a long time. The workshop organizers invited scholars
(sociologists, bioethicists, etc.) to reflect on the ethical implications of
using CRISPR/Cas9, a procedure for altering and editing genes, on
human embryos. The occasion was that a Chinese researcher, He Jankui,
had used this technique on human embryos to 'give' them the genetic
variant associated with HIV immunity.[2] Several talks at the workshop
engaged with whether embryo editing, using CRISPR/Cas9, was less
ethical than embryo selection.

Embryo selection, or preimplantation genetic testing, has existed
for decades. It means creating several embryos *in vitro* and performing
genetic testing on them. Prospective parents can opt for this procedure
if they risk transmitting a genetic mutation to their offspring. The
embryos that are found to carry the genetic mutation are discarded.
Only embryo(s) free of the mutation are transferred to the prospective
mother's uterus. In the case of embryo editing, which CRISPR/Cas9 has
made feasible, it could, in principle, be possible to create one embryo
and 'fix' the genetic mutation in that embryo. Each approach has its
benefits. Embryo selection is a tried technique and is less invasive as it
does not require changing the genetic code. However, at least one of the
embryos must be free of the mutation, which is sometimes impossible.
It is also impossible to insert new genes into the embryo: you must work
with the genetic material of the persons from whom the sperm or egg
originated. CRISPR/Cas9 could, in principle, be used to 'fix' genetic
material that is not already available in one of the embryos. Hence, new
genetic material can be added to the embryo.

From a conceptual point of view, there may be another difference
between the two techniques that some presenters deemed relevant.
First, in the case of embryo selection, the embryos that do have the
mutation associated with the disease will be discarded. Throwing away
embryos may be unacceptable for people who believe that embryos are
potential or actual human persons. In the case of CRISPR, in principle,
only one embryo is created, which is then 'fixed'. So theoretically, no

---

2   Although this is not entirely what happened. He introduced a change in the DNA
     that he hoped emulated the behaviour of the gene that is responsible for HIV
     resistance in some people.

embryos would have to be discarded. I say 'theoretically' because the fact remains that embryos may perish spontaneously *in vitro*, so the procedure could have to be repeated several times. Moreover, many embryos will have been discarded during the experimental phase to develop both techniques. Nevertheless, when in 2016, the first so-called three-parent baby was born, it was rumoured that the prospective parents chose nuclear transfer ('three-parent baby' technique) rather than embryo selection to avoid the destruction of multiple embryos. The 'three-parent baby' technique can be used when the prospective mother risks transferring a mitochondrial disease to the child. The technique implies that the nucleus of the prospective mother's egg is inserted in an enucleated oocyte from a donor. Thus, the mitochondria from the donor are used. For this technique, embryo selection is, in many cases, possible. The first baby conceived in this way was born in 2016 in Mexico. The story goes that the (presumably Catholic) prospective parents chose this method so that no embryos would be discarded.

As I have stated before, the distinction between choosing an embryo with 'better' genes or changing an embryo so that it has other genes seems relevant. This distinction is relevant regardless of the opinion of ethicists about the embryo's status and whether they can accept that some embryos might be discarded. In the case of embryo selection, so the argument goes, you are choosing one future person over another. Even if we do not consider an *in vitro* embryo a person, the hope is that it will eventually become one. In the case of embryo editing, we are not choosing one future person over another. However, we are changing their genetic makeup so they will not develop a specific condition. Suppose we accept that genetic modification will give the future person a better life because they will be free of a debilitating condition. There may even be a moral duty to do so in that case. Therein, some people argue, lies the difference with embryo selection. In the latter case, we do not only increase the likelihood of a future person leading a life free of a known condition, but we are also choosing which embryo to apply this to and, in doing so, choose one future person over another. Chance is replaced by choice. Some ethicists, such as Julian Savulescu, argue that if we can select one future person over another and this one person has less chance of developing a disorder, we have a moral duty to do so (Savulescu, 2001; Savulescu and Kahane, 2009). However, if we consider

Parfit's remarks, we may also wonder for whom this action would be better. After all, the embryos that were not chosen had nothing to lose in the first place. We do not decide whether the embryos will have a specific disorder. The discarded embryos will merely not be born. If you consider being born better than not being born,[3] there is no reason why picking the embryo without the mutation is better for the embryo not picked. The notable exception would be if the disorder selected against would result in life below the threshold of what is worth living. Such a threshold is difficult to define, as this may imply predicting what might be, by definition, unpredictable. However, it is difficult to say that not picking an embryo without the mutation harms the embryo with the mutation: the former future human would not come into existence. For the latter embryo, in an embryo selection procedure, the life with the mutation is simply the only one available, and such a life may be preferable to no life at all. In the case of embryo editing, the situation is different. Here, the argument goes, we are changing the person the embryo will become. Here the choice is between having a life without the disease-causing mutation or a life with the disease-causing mutation. If we consider the question of whether happiness or well-being depends upon whether someone is susceptible to a genetic disease or not, this seems relevant. If we do not remove the genetic mutation, provided that we can do this safely and efficiently, we may be negligent and cause this future person unnecessary harm.

The non-identity problem has puzzled reproductive ethicists for decades, to the extent that some people just choose to ignore it. After all, many of us would like to argue that if it is indeed possible to pick a 'better' embryo, or at least an embryo that will be spared a devastating genetic disease, then we must do so. However, in this workshop on the borders of Lake Geneva, the non-identity problem was used in several talks to argue for or against embryo selection or embryo editing. It is not my aim here to comment on the ethical conclusions or even to question the use of the non-identity problem in reproductive ethics. There may very well be good reasons why non-identity matters. Instead, I would like to reflect on which basis the identity problem occurs. It seems that,

---

3   Of course, we should not take for granted the fact that being born is actually better than not being born, as is argued by David Benatar in *Better Never to Have Been* (Benatar, 2008).

like Derek Parfit, many ethicists thought that what happens at conception is indeed unique (Parfit, 1984). It is where an individual starts existing. Even secular ethicists, regardless of their opinion on the status of the embryo, think that causing potential harm or benefit to one embryo and not to another is relevant, as it is this embryo that eventually becomes a person. There is a period after conception when the embryo could still split into monozygous twins. This time frame ends around the fourteenth day post-conception, when something called the primitive streak forms. For some, this moment also has moral significance, as it is deemed to be the moment when the embryo is considered an individual (Steinbock, 1992). Interestingly, the discussions about the embryo's moral status centre around the embryo's characteristics. Some would argue that, as it has all the potential to develop into a human being, it already has dignity and should be treated with respect. Others state that such an early embryo is just a bunch of cells and, therefore, cannot have dignity or moral standing. However, most reproductive ethicists do not deny that an *in vitro* embryo has an identity. Granted, everyone alive today originated from a specific embryo. What is less clear is that this type of numerical identity matters morally.

I can think of two reasons why this would be the case. First, it is possible that what counts is the numerical identity. So regardless of whether we can imagine that a given embryo can develop into different people with different personalities if it were to grow up in other circumstances in parallel universes, it is trivial that one embryo will be one person in the same universe. It is strange, though, that this merely numerical fact carries so much normative weight in discussions about harm to persons or non-persons, and it may be worth reflecting somewhat longer on why this is so. Scholars probably consider it relevant here that this embryo has a unique combination of genes that will remain the same during its lifespan. Even if the embryo *in vitro* per se is nothing but a bunch of cells, it already contains its essence, the (nuclear) DNA. Therefore, we may think that if we pick embryo A over embryo B, these will have different identities, even if they were raised in the same circumstances. Furthermore, what we think is essential for normative conclusions here is the unique genetic combination of each embryo. However, if that is the case, it complicates the discussion of CRISPR even further, even without considering epigenetics. If we edit an embryo to avoid a particular congenital disorder, we, in fact, also change its genetic makeup. Rather than 'curing' an embryo, we create a different person. If genetics is the decisive factor in identity, this may also be ethically relevant.

With these reflections, it is not my aim to draw a specific conclusion or argue one way or another. Ethical arguments for and against particular techniques that refer to the non-identity problem are often relatively dry and technical and have ideas that are hard to waylay. It is important to keep questioning the basis on which these arguments rest and which we often take for granted. What is an identity, and why would numerical identity matter so much? Maybe the importance we attributed to genetic identity suggests a preformationist view on identity and personhood at its heart. If we think about our identity, we think about something that is both stable and develops over time. Perhaps a Waddingtonian landscape is a good metaphor with stability and plasticity to adapt. This means that what is relevant in discussions about future well-being and responsibility in reproductive ethics should not only hinge on genes remaining the same but also consider the entire development of an organism, from conception until death, and encompass all its experiences and chance encounters. When we think about embryos, the future child we feel responsible for is not available yet. Interventions that change a person's possible experiences may be more identity-affecting than a combination of genes.

Perhaps a truly developmental perspective on identity would allow us to forego these technical discussions on numerical identities and focus on other things, such as the importance of experience and context for identity. Maybe it is time for reproductive ethics to question its reliance on the primacy of genes for arguments. My gut feeling is that this would open up new perspectives beyond focusing on what happens *in vitro*. Nevertheless, I will leave this discussion and its potential implications for now. To fully appreciate the importance of chance and experiences, an epigenetic or developmental view of life may not yield the entire picture. The environment itself may still be a deterministic prison. As I have already hinted, epigenetics may demonstrate that we are open systems all the way into our molecules. This realisation opens up possibilities to see life differently.

In the last chapter of the 2003 collection *Cycles of Contingency*, Cor van der Weele states that 'DST (Developmental Systems Theory) and ethics in their present forms are clearly distinguished as normative enterprises, or, if you prefer, are worlds apart' (Oyama, Griffiths and Gray, 2003). As I aim to bring bioethics and systems thinking in biology together, I dedicated this first part to describing the relationship between science and philosophy and ethics. I used the case of Macchiarini to argue that philosophers and ethicists should be included in scientific research projects from their inception onwards. They can function as benevolent gadflies. As gadflies, their task is to demand conceptual clarity and explanations of ideas that scientists may take for granted. In the final two chapters of Part One, I described how ethicists sometimes take concepts, such as identity, for granted. Given the sizeable existing corpus in bioethics on the ethics of genes, I spent some time explaining some of the concepts and ideas that permeate the discussion. Starting from the original meaning of 'epigenesis' and tracking this through Waddington's epigenetic landscape, I described how these findings suggest a dynamic view of biology that we do not always acknowledge in current bioethical discussions on genes and genetic technologies. In the next part of the book, I will describe a view of life that stresses historicity, indeterminacy, and chance encounters. I will argue that, given the entanglement of organism and milieu, to understand and appreciate the phenomena of life, how life is experienced may be as important as understanding its mechanisms.

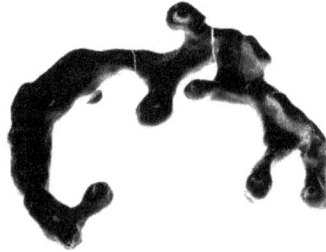

Rapchiy

What are the hidden designs of a mind-brain dualism supporting commercial brain data measuring device?

From: Synaptic Morphing: hidden brain reader designs transformed from paper sketch into ceramics.

Photo by Bartaku, 2017.[4]

---

4   In the period 2016–2018, at various public events visitors were invited to place a broken EMOTIV Epoc device on their head, with a thin sheet of paper in between. Another visitor traced the outlines of the device with a pen. At each event a set of drawings or 'hidden designs' was generated. These were transformed into 3D ceramic sculptural pieces using varying techniques and matter. See the chapter 'Synaptic Morphing' in Vandeput, B (Bartaku) 2021, *Baroa belaobara*: berryapple (diss.), pp. 167–197, Aalto University, Espoo, https://research.aalto.fi/en/publications/baroa-belaobara-berryapple

PART TWO: CHANCE AND CREATIVITY

In which I argue for chance encounters, for making worlds and being made by worlds

Intelligence is a complex instinct which hasn't yet fully matured. The idea is that instinctive activity is always natural and useful. A million years will pass, the instinct will mature, and we will cease making the mistakes which are probably an integral part of intelligence. And then, if anything in the universe changes, we will happily become extinct-again, precisely because we've lost the art of making mistakes, that is, trying various things not prescribed by a rigid code.

– Roadside Picnic, Arkady & Boris Strugatski
(Strugatsky, Strugatsky and Bormashenko, 2012, p. 130)

Man has long been aware that his World has a tendency to fall apart. Tools wear out, fishing nets need repair, roofs leak, iron rusts, wood decays, loved ones die.

– Van Rensselaer Potter (Rensselaer Potter, 1971, p. 56)

The Earth produces as many things as she is capable of producing: There is not such a thing as 'man' but there are 'men', no 'human' but 'humans'. There is no such thing as a 'cat'. There are, instead, jaguars, lions, ocelots, tigers, leopards and so on. The world is a fulsome place.

– Viola F. Cordova (Cordova, 2007, p. 106)

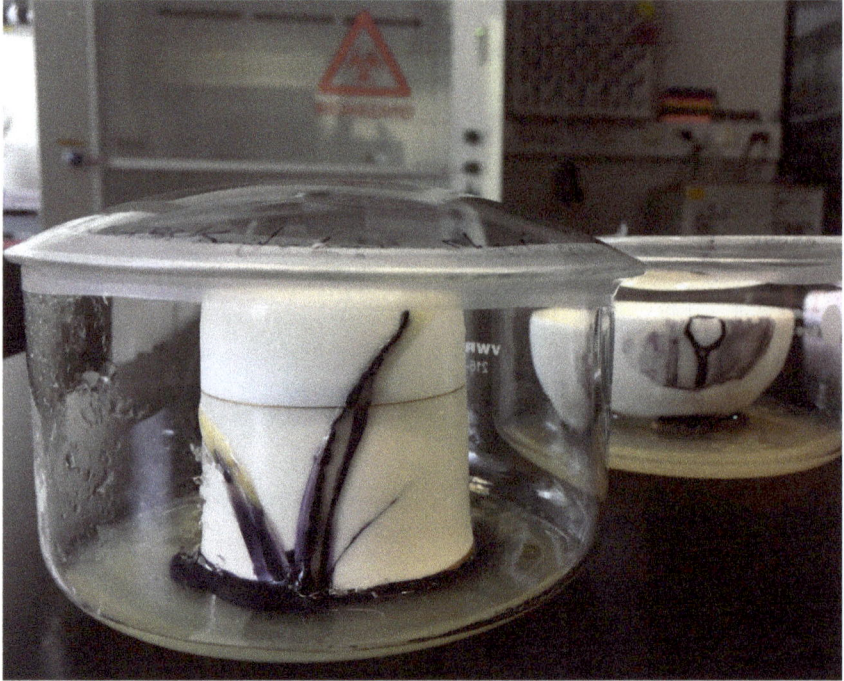

Repairing a crack by growing a scar.
From: Ceramic Scar Tissue. Artistic research of the concept of healing by proposing
micro-biological Kin Tsugi.
Photo by Christina Stadlbauer, 2018[1]

---

1   Ceramic Scar Tissue, ongoing since 2018. Work was shown at the exhibition
     "Narratives of Imperfection" in Helsinki and Tokyo, 2019. https://www.research
     catalogue.net/view/761499/761500

In Part One, I described some aspects of the relationship between bioethics, philosophy, and science. By explaining that bioethics and philosophy of science should join forces, I illustrated how and why this would help scientists to weed out pointless or even dangerous practices and yet keep science adventurous and capable of leading to better futures. I continued by describing how bioethics should critically engage with science and reflect on conceptual schemes that are both readily assumed and in popular media. I zoomed in on the normative implications of the nature-nurture distinction and the concept of the gene. Emphasizing a developmental view on life, Epigenetics enlightened us on how we, as bioethicists, tackled questions surrounding genetics. It may suggest a way out of determinism and reductionism. At the same time, there is a danger that epigenetics does not resolve the old dichotomies. A focus on environmental or even epigenetic effects may indeed in itself be deterministic.

This chapter will delve deeper into the relationship between science, life, and bioethics. Van Rensselaer Potter was convinced that biology should inform bioethics. This idea, for him, meant that, ultimately, the goal of bioethics is the survival of humankind. We have to take what we know about biology to formulate such ethics. Interestingly, Potter had a specific idea about life that he thought should be the basis of bioethics. He was committed to a view of life that acknowledges the importance of order and disorder. He admits that humans do not tolerate a lack of order very well. Science and religion try to set the 'ground rules' for the organization of the universe; in that respect, they are the same. Genetic determinism and reductionism are ultimately a symptom of the search for order. Nevertheless, as I will demonstrate later in the chapter, Potter believed that disorder is as fundamental as order if we want to understand life and reality. Disorder allows for creativity and freedom. As bioethicists, we must deal with chaos and unpredictability as much as predictability. However, ultimately, disorder also will enable us to make choices and choose between different paths.

In what follows, I will describe the ideas of philosophers and scientists that have thought about life, (dis)order and creativity. These authors are not usually part of the traditional bioethics curriculum. As a bioethicist, my task is to waver between questions regarding life and survival on the one hand and concrete analyses and even guidelines on the other. This position implies being inspired by different traditions and translating these traditions into a language that is acceptable to people.

6. A Dog Is a Dog Is a Dog

Of Nature and Values

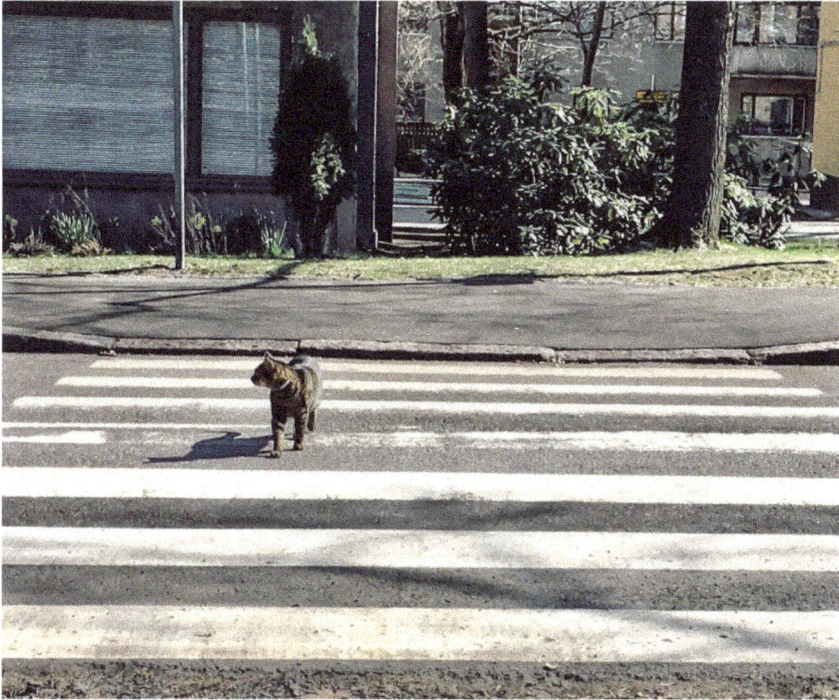

Mr Pussovitch, most probably the only free-ranging cat in the streets of Helsinki.
How to provide a non-hierarchical co-existing with other-than-humans.
Photo, Bartaku, 2020[2]

---

2   Hieronymus Pussovitch has chosen his human companions on the streets of Brussels
    in 2013. Then he relocated with them to Helsinki in 2016, where he has been living
    until September 2022. He is free ranging and very experienced with traffic and its
    rules. He mostly reaches the other side of the streets by walking on the zebra crossings.
    The picture was taken during one of his regular walks with his human companion.

   https://doi.org/10.11647/OBP.0320.06

In his book *Bioethics, A Bridge to the Future*, Van Rensselaer Potter explicitly advocates for biology-inspired ethics (Potter, 1971). He dedicates the book's first chapter to describing a view on biology and asserting that this view should be at the heart of bioethics inquiry. His view is surprisingly similar to the more recent views I described in the previous chapter. At the same time, the rise and popularity of cybernetics in the mid-twentieth century is still pervasive in *Bioethics: Bridge to the Future*, in which he calls human beings error-prone cybernetic machines. (Potter, 1971) Nevertheless, the machine that is a human being is not merely a simple mechanism. Instead, Potter states, 'Man is an adaptive control system with elements of disorder built into every hierarchical level'. This disorder is built into every level of functioning, from the DNA to how our mind functions. In fact, according to Potter, it is because there is disorder that there is novelty and freedom. After all, we can make mistakes, introduce novelty into our lives, and learn in hindsight. Our behaviour is not merely the behaviour of an automaton. We can 'depart from the established norm'. For Potter, this is specifically so for human organisms, who have 'more opportunity for the exercise of the individual free will than other forms'. He concludes that this is the starting point for bioethics:

> The idea that man's survival is a problem in economics and political science is a myth that assumes that man is free or could be free from the forces of nature. These disciplines help to tell us what men want, but it may require biology to tell what man can have, i.e., what constraints operate in the relationship between mankind and the natural World. Bioethics would attempt to balance cultural appetites against physiological needs in terms of public policy. A desirable cultural adaptation in our society would be a more widespread knowledge of the nature and limitations of all kinds of adaptation.
>
> Bioethics, as I envision it, would attempt to generate wisdom, the knowledge of how to use knowledge for social good from a realistic knowledge of man's biological nature and of the biological World. To me, realistic knowledge of man is a knowledge that includes his role as an adaptive control system with built-in error tendencies. This mechanistic view, which combines reductionist and holistic elements, would be totally incapable of generating wisdom unless supplemented with both a humanistic and an ecological outlook. [...] The present World is dominated by military policy and by an overemphasis on production of material goods. Neither of these enterprises have given any thought to

the basic facts of biology. An urgent task for Bioethics is to seek biological agreements at the international level. (Rensselaer Potter, 1971, p. 26)

Hence, Potter argues, there should be a rapprochement between humanities scholars and biology. Such harmonization does not seek to make biology and biotechnology more ethical but necessitates that humanities should start from biologically sound ideas. They should be informed by biology. Only in this way will humanities and biological sciences succeed in what must be their most pressing aim: to guarantee the survival of humankind.

In *A Bridge to the Future*, Van Rensselaer Potter claims that 'Man's survival may depend on ethics based on biological knowledge; hence Bioethics' (Rensselaer Potter, 1971, p. 1). In his 1988 book, *Global Bioethics*, Potter describes how C. H. Waddington influenced his biology-inspired bioethics (Potter, 1988). According to Potter, Waddington was 'a bioethicist before the word was invented, a man concerned with the need to develop ethical theory in the light of biological knowledge'. (Potter, 1988, p. 2). In papers such as *The Relations Between Ethics and Science*, Waddington argues how the Good is dependent on the characteristics of the World in general (Waddington, 1944). This idea seems straightforward, yet at the same time, it feels like blasphemy. The naturalistic fallacy is one of the fallacies we often teach students in bioethics classes. One cannot just read ethical norms from biological findings. We tell them. Potter was aware of this false reasoning and quotes from Conrad Waddington's *The Ethical Animal* to refute the idea that ethics cannot be based on biology:

> We can, with perfect logical consistency, conceive of an aim or principle of policy which, while not in itself in its essence an ethical rule, would enable us to judge between different ethical rules. It is for such a principle that I am searching, and which I claim to be discoverable in the notion which I have referred to as 'biological wisdom'... To a theory which attempted to discover a criterion for judging between ethical systems, the refutation of the naturalistic fallacy would be largely beside the point. (Potter, 1988, p. 5)

The above ideas tie in with the more general tendency of human beings to look for values in nature, as is comprehensively explored in Lorraine Daston's excellent book *Against Nature* (Daston, 2019). She states, 'the urge to seek order and to represent is intrinsic to human rationality, and the human kind of reason is the only kind of reason we have' (ibid.). Still, the idea of bioethics based on biological principles seems naïve and perhaps even dangerous. We can think about the dangers of taking the 'is' to 'ought' step too readily. More work and extra steps need to be done to consider what ought to be done based on *what is the case* than merely reading it from empirical data. Consider assumptions regarding the role of women in society. Suppose that our ancestors had a traditional role pattern where a woman stayed home and a man would go hunting. Such an empirical finding would imply that it is good that women stay home, even if their ambitions lay elsewhere. Another example is the argument that is sometimes given against vegetarianism. Undoubtedly, human beings are omnivorous, so the argument goes. We must only look at our teeth to have proof of that. Alternatively, consider the statements regarding the 'naturalness' of certain types of sexuality. Undoubtedly, these arguments do much harm and demonstrate that we cannot just 'read' what is good from what is. Nevertheless, what is the relationship between ethics and nature? Did Van Rensselaer Potter make a capital mistake when he thought that ethics should be inspired by (a specific view on) biology?

The relationship between ethics and biology has been puzzling me for a long time, specifically when considering human relationships with other-than-human animals. When I was a master's student in Applied Ethics, I wrote a paper on the ethics of companion animals (Hens, 2009). More specifically, I focussed on the relationship human beings have with dogs. I challenged accounts where this relationship was seen as instrumentalization or domination, as in Yi-Fu Tuan's seminal work *Dominance and Affection* (Tuan, 1984). Animal rights activists such as Gary Francione think that our relationship with companion animals is one of property (Francione, 2012). To the law, companion animals are our property. However, from a particular deontological perspective, they cannot be. The fact that they are de facto property implies that companion animals, preferably, should not exist. Using the words of the late philosopher Tom Regan, an animal is not a means to an end (Potter, 1988). Therefore, we should not keep pets, even if we treat them well, love them and care for them. Deep ecologists, who consider nature intrinsically valuable, regardless of its use to human beings, such as Paul Shepard, have sometimes argued that there is something wrong with our relationship with companion animals (Shepard, 1997). Companion animals are *Ersatz*. Some would even say they are a travesty of wild animals. In this view, dogs are a watered-down version of wolves, and we are mistaken if we think that our relationship with dogs is somehow a modern version of more primordial contact with nature. In my Master's paper, I looked at relatively recent ideas about the origins of our relationship with dogs (Hens, 2009). Archaeological and anthropological evidence suggests that our relationship with dogs is far more complex than merely one of taming and dominion. The canine origin story of a Pleistocene child who found a wolf puppy that became a helpful hunting partner, as Konrad Lorenz told it, is wrong. If we look at semi-wild dogs in different parts of the world, we can see that stray dogs often follow human tribes and live on their leftovers. Recent scholars have thus suggested that dogs have, to some degree, domesticated themselves. The wolves that were less afraid than their peers started following early humans and their settlements. These tamer wolves had access to different food sources than their cousins, who preferred to stay away from human beings. In this way, wolves became dogs even before people kept them as companions. They had domesticated themselves. The relationship between humans and dogs is thus one of *coevolution*.

I thought at the time that this was relevant to the ethics argument. We cannot just assume that the relationship with dogs is one of dominion or that dogs are degenerate wolves. Their existence is proof that natural and cultural history are not separate things. Arguments referencing an original wild wolf that was then dominated are misguided. In conclusion, our relationship with companion dogs is *sui generis*. It is unique and worthwhile. At the same time, the fact that dogs are to some extent at our mercy and that we have such power to control their lives in all aspects, from the food they eat and the reproductive options they have, suggests that we have an even more outstanding obligation to care for them. The article about dogs was my first scholarly article in applied ethics. Since then, I have become much more familiar with metaethics, and I started wondering whether I had been mistaken. I cringe if people use hypotheses from evolutionary psychology and evolutionary biology to defend status quos, such as the position of women in a patriarchal society. Maybe I was making the same mistake here.

Historically, the relationship between empirical facts and norms has been discussed in philosophical discussions between ethical (or moral) naturalists and non-naturalists. Ethical naturalists state that what is morally good can be discovered by looking at the scientific data and be logically deduced from that data. For example, Peter Railton says that an act is morally good only if the deed is done by an entirely rational and informed subject (a subject that has 'looked at the data' and has an objective view of the world)(Railton, 1986). This need not only be data from the exact sciences. For Railton, we should also take the social point of view and include all involved interests. As such, moral statements are objective; they can be 'fact checked'.

The most well-known name associated with ethical non-naturalism is G. E. Moore (1873–1958). He states that if moral goodness would coincide with a natural characteristic (for example, what is good is pleasurable), then the question of whether a specific act that increases pleasure is good is meaningless because the answer would be, per definition, positive (Moore, 1933). Hence, the question would make as little sense as asking whether bachelors are unmarried (Moore, 1993). For Moore, however, the question about the goodness of acts does make sense. It is essential for morality that we ask the question. Hence, goodness is a fundamental, separate characteristic that cannot be directly deduced from natural facts. It follows that the properties of goodness cannot be defined but can only be shown and grasped. Goodness is what our moral intuitions point to, not what we can imply from empirical data.

The task of the bioethicist is to give concrete answers to ethical problems arising from new technologies and progress in biomedical sciences. To do that, we must consider scientific facts as part of moral deliberation. It seems wrong to only take into account our intuitions. For example, people may intuitively feel that genetically modifying plants are no good (the 'yuk feeling'). Intuition varies from person to person and is influenced by everyone's environment and experiences. Especially in a field like bioethics, it is crucial to look at and thoroughly understand the scientific facts and advantages that such technologies may yield. However, this does not mean we can merely deduce good and bad from a risk-benefit analysis. Evaluative judgments unavoidably creep into such risk-benefit analysis itself. Evaluating whether a specific use of technology is morally good requires something more from us than a mere balancing exercise. At the same time, that does not mean that our ontological commitments are not the basis of our ethical reasoning. To go back to the previous section, if we think about the possibility of changing an embryo's genes for the best, we are committed to a view of the world in which such alterations can change a life course for the best. Rather than extracting solutions to ethical dilemmas from reality, a commitment to naturalism may also mean ensuring that our conceptual schemes are consistent. Hence, I think Van Rensselaer Potter was right that ethics, which has a primary aim to ensure a liveable future, should be guided by the most recent findings in biology and physics. Ezequiel Di Paulo and Hanne De Jaegher have described this beautifully in the article Enactive Ethics: Difference Becoming Participation (Di Paolo and De Jaegher, 2021). They argue that any dualism between ethics and science is only relevant if we have a reductionist and mechanistic perspective on human biology. From such a perspective, empirical data are things to 'read out'. Di Paulo and De Jaegher argue that care and normativity are grounded in forms of life: we care about the world we live in. I will reflect on how this ties in with care ethics in the fourth part of this book. A truly biological bioethics is thus committed to an ontology of becoming, of change. It is, at the same time, backwards-informed and forward-looking. Our biological and cultural history tells us something about our choices for the future. We are neither determined by our history nor doomed to repeat it, but history defines our current situation and dictates that we must move forward. There is no going back to a more pristine state. In the spirit of Donna Haraway, we must stay with the trouble that is our world and decide what we can do next to maintain ourselves in this troubled world.

Donna Haraway is such a philosopher who, inspired by her relationship with her dogs, thinks about nature and culture, the nature of 'nature'. She also offers a way out of my doubts regarding the ethics of dog keeping (Haraway, 2007, 2013). For Haraway, dogs and companion animals are not degenerated versions of creatures that lived in a lost paradise. In her ontology, there is no space for such dualities. Dogs and humans are equivalent because we incorporate the wild and the tamed, nature and culture. They cannot be but closely linked to humanity; otherwise, they would not be dogs. However, it would be wrong to see that as a bad thing. Like humans and dogs, there is no pristine nature to return to or take as a template of how things should be. We should think about our collective history and the future we want for dogs as dogs. This means staying with the trouble of many uncomfortable truths about companion animals, such as the control we have over their bodies and reproductive systems in order for them to live in households sustainably. Nevertheless, staying with the trouble does not mean we take this as morally good without further ado. It means accepting the complexities of the choices we make.

7. A Process Ontology for Bioethics

Prehensions and Actual Occasions

In the previous sections, I have described how we can look at the phenomenon of life from a developmental perspective. This perspective can free us from the fiction that who we are is somehow fixed at conception. It also puts question marks around the idea that genes can predict behaviour. Organisms develop in close interaction with the environment that they also create. Organisms have a history, and epigenetics makes biology, to some extent, a historical science. The idea that an organism is dynamically co-constructed by the environment is widely accepted. However, some would argue that this co-construction can be known and calculated by taking comprehensive data about genes and the environment into account. They believe that it is still possible to predict its future.

In what follows, I will delve deeper into some theories by physicists, chemists, biologists, and philosophers to investigate concepts of uncertainty and indeterminacy. I do so because I believe that the topics we choose (genes, hacking evolution etc.) are often influenced by how we think the world functions. As bioethicists, we take over much of the ways things are discussed in scientific papers. However, as I have argued, such views are sometimes inspired by a mechanistic worldview, especially in medical science. Many proponents of physics and economic sciences have given up such a mechanistic worldview. I aim to make some of their thoughts relevant to bioethics in what follows. To do so, I first want to describe the worldview I think will become predominant in the 21st century. I will use the ideas of thinkers such as Alfred North

 https://doi.org/10.11647/OBP.0320.07

Whitehead, Ilya Prigogine, Isabelle Stengers, Stuart Kauffman, Karen Barad, and Donna Haraway. These thinkers are not the ones that are commonly used in bioethics papers. This omission may be due to a clash of traditions— much bioethics is steeped in the analytic tradition of using conceptual analysis and references to empirical data. We usually write argumentative books and papers with clarity. The authors I have mentioned are speculative: they suggest new ways of looking at reality and life. It must be said that they do so from a scientific starting point: they are often scientists who are also well-versed in philosophy. I know that by emphasizing these thinkers' scientific background, I am residing here to an argument from authority. Sometimes, such statements, although flawed, are all there is left to make a point. When I presented an early version of the ideas that inspired me to write this book at a conference full of bioethicists, one well-known bioethicist talked to me during the break and told me, 'Kristien, you still have to stick to the science'.

Nevertheless, the ideas I presented were the ideas of scientists. Moreover, I would contend that the gene-centric worldview, often considered science-based and prevalent in bioethics, is becoming obsolete. In a previous chapter, I referred to the Lake Geneva Conference on CRISPR/Cas9 on the ethics of changing the genetic makeup o human in vitro embryos. In many talks, people took it for granted that, in principle, it will eventually be possible to use this technology in embryos to avoid congenital and other diseases and, as many assumed, to alter other traits of individuals. What we need to think about, as bioethicists, is whether it is desirable for this possibility to become a reality or not. I would contend that several aspects of the underlying viewpoints are problematic. These viewpoints include the idea that risks related to genetic technologies can never be objectively weighed against one another. They also believe that traits and behaviours are primarily genetic and that, ultimately, we will be able to predict things like intelligence. While many contemporary scientists would argue against that, I perceive that such assumptions are still taken for granted in popular science media and grant proposals alike.

I will present the views of scientists confronted with questions that cannot be answered within the standard frame of reference of specific science. They seek to understand reality and life differently. Their common thought is that the reality of being is primarily characterized by processes rather than governed by determinism and predictability. What matters in such an approach are relations, encounters, and choices rather than adherence to strict laws. Alfred North Whitehead is the philosopher and mathematician who is first and foremost associated with this kind of thinking and has inspired biologists, new materialists, and theologists alike. His magnum opus, *Process and Reality*, is not an easy nut to crack (Whitehead, 2010). Its speculative nature seems to get in the way of any practical application of his thinking, for example, in applied ethics.

Moreover, many secular bioethicists and analytic philosophers associate him with theology, and God has a prominent role in his thinking. As a secular bioethicist, I understand this worry. However, I also concluded while reading the book that we do not need to accept a traditional vision of God or even accept the role Whitehead has assigned to God in his work to appreciate what he is trying to tell us. In what follows, I will try to convey the overall gist of his thinking—or at least what I believe may be relevant—for bioethics.[1] The following text is heavily inspired by Ronny Desmet's fascinating presentation to my research team. He introduces us to the life and thinking of Alfred North Whitehead andwe had illuminating discussions about how to make this relevant to our research. I understand that there is a common sentiment that trying to sum up great thinkers in a few simplistic paragraphs seems blasphemous. I also honestly believe that if we want to tackle 21st-century problems, we need to integrate interesting thoughts from many different exciting thinkers. In this respect, for an applied ethicist like myself, the possibility to avail oneself of titbits of exciting information is paramount. Those not interested in some of the more technical details of Whitehead's thinking may skip the following paragraph and jump to the next one, where I try to make some of his thinking relevant to Bioethics.

Alfred North Whitehead (1861–1947) was trained as a mathematician and philosopher. He is perhaps best known for his book with Bertrand Russel, *Principia Mathematica* (Whitehead and Russell, 1927). As a

---

1 In 2019, colleagues and I had a book club on Whitehead. We were greatly helped by discussing the work with Ronny Desmet, Whitehead scholar and co-author of the Stanford Encyclopaedia of Philosophy entry on Whitehead. Before tacking *Process and Reality* itself, I read John Cobb's *Whitehead Word Book*, which was of great help(Cobb and Jr., 2015).

mathematician and philosopher, he was influenced by Maxwell's theory of electromagnetism. His philosophy is one of relations, of *processes*. It gave rise to what we now call process philosophy and process theology—although we can trace back process thinking to ancient Greeks such as Heraclitus. In Whitehead's view, nature is a tissue of internally related events. These internally connected events affect one another. He is opposed to a mechanistic world view, where we can see nature as a clock composed of gear wheels that work together but can be considered separately. What are these events, and on what level should we consider them? Reading Whitehead's *Process and Reality* means getting to know a wonderful world of things like prehensions, actual entities and actual occasions (Whitehead, 2010). His ontology is an event ontology. An event, or actual occasion, has a time dimension: It is on a historical route incorporating all the previous routes and outside influences. However, an actual occasion is not deterministically defined by its history. There is an element of experience, of evaluating what has happened before. Facts from the past do not determine the present, but they cast a shadow of potentialities. Integrating them in an actual occasion means considering these potentialities. This experience is called prehension. It is the moment an elementary particle evaluates and integrates previous occasions. Hence, because of this moment of prehension, the future cannot be automatically deduced from the past. There is a moment of indeterminacy, or even choice, in the act of integration.

At the same time, what is in the past is a given and cannot be changed. There is a real arrow in time, something I will talk a little bit more about later on. You may wonder what kind of things these actual occasions are. Who is doing the prehension? Originally, Whitehead described this event ontology in the context of elementary particles—the electron, more specifically. It is the electron that has a history and an undetermined future. The electron evaluates and prehends. Later, Whitehead will say that this description applies to all layers of the universe, from electrons to plants, other-than-human animals and human animals.

Electrons that can experience things are a strange idea. Is Whitehead assuming that electrons, and, by extension, all matter, are conscious? Discussions about panpsychism, the idea that all things have a mind, are very lively in the 21st century. However, I do not think we need to consider Whitehead's description as one of panpsychism. Although Whitehead agrees that from the electron to the human being, they can all experience things, this experience is not synonymous with consciousness. For him, consciousness is an emergent property related to how sophisticated the integration, the prehension, is. Everything that makes up reality can experience these possibilities from past occasions and integrate and evaluate them. Nevertheless, in the case of consciousness and conscious being, this integration is related to the sophistication of the integration. Consciousness is an advanced form of experience not present in all entities. Still, the suggestion that electrons might feel or experience stuff may sound weird. It seems to be consistent with some phenomena that have been described in quantum mechanics. Phenomena such as spooky action at a distance may be difficult to explain without assuming some experiential property of elementary particles. At the same time, such ideas contradict our deepest intuitions.

Whitehead describes a universe that is constantly in evolution, that continually progresses, a creative universe, to say in the words of Stuart Kauffman (Kauffman, 2016). This creativity does not imply a universe of unbound and endless possibilities. In evaluating and choosing one way or another, our options are limited. They depend on the circumstances and what has happened in the past. I would contend they also depend on the things and creatures one encounters and relates to. It is an act of integration to bring these together and create a liveable future. Whitehead suggests that history progresses as events incorporate their past and create something new. However, this does not mean that this progress is necessary for the good. There is much leeway for choice, but choices are not always good. We may be headed for catastrophe if wrong decisions are made. Some scholars, such as Isabelle Stengers, have taken Whiteheadian thought and have used it to reflect on the environmental crisis (Stengers, 2020). There is no guarantee that humanity will turn out all right in the end. Not even Whitehead's God can do that.

I think it is possible to appreciate Whitehead's world without acknowledging the existence of a God. Maybe the electron with experiences is a bridge too far for many of us. We intuitively make a strict distinction between dead matter and alive organisms. I shall describe another thinker, Karen Barad, who challenges this distinction. At the same time, Whitehead's ontology fits a developmental perspective on life very well. Conrad Waddington, who invented the image of the epigenetic landscape, knew Whitehead and his ideas. Epigenetics and the epigenetic landscape point to a historical approach to organisms. Such a historical approach is one of adapting to new circumstances and, simultaneously, trying to maintain one's own in changing circumstances. Epigenetics is often said to inscribe an organism's biography into its cells: we are what we have experienced. It all fits well with a Whiteheadian approach, and the thinkers I will describe next can all, to some extent, be considered process thinkers.

Whiteheadian Fallacies

I want to illustrate the relevance of Whitehead and what he can bring to bioethics using his ideas on science. For Whitehead, contrary to what we may intuitively assume, philosophers (and scientists) should be wary of abstractions. Striving for abstractions should not be our ultimate goal. This idea aligns with Whitehead's event ontology, as I have described above: reality is to be conceived as an entangled maze of relationships, where new events incorporate the past in a non-deterministic way. Elementary particles are historical trajectories of events. Such an ontology implies that it is most important to understand reality in its concreteness if we want to know anything about it.

For Whitehead, the concrete is always more 'true' than the abstract. This insight is utterly relevant for bioethical and other methodologies. In my research, I have always wondered why quantitative research is often considered more scientific and closer to the truth than qualitative research. Quantitative research is usually done with surveys and includes abstractions such as the mean and the deviation. Qualitative researchers, on the contrary, look for idiosyncrasies and context-specific experiences. Qualitative research is not about what most subjects may feel or think. I have done much such research, and sometimes participants ask me, what do you learn from this? Why is my peculiar experience relevant to you? Would it not be better to survey many respondents with a specific condition X if we try to find out what condition X is? Qualitative researchers submitting their work to peer-reviewed journals have met with questions about their limited sample size by reviewers unaccustomed to this kind of research. I think Whitehead would disagree with the preference for quantitative data, and so do I.

Insight into concrete situations is as scientific as generalizations based on many data. However, I also acknowledge that we cannot do without abstractions and generalizations in science. In the given example of researching 'condition X', it would most likely be impossible to investigate each instance as a case in its own right, even if it would give a more comprehensive understanding of certain phenomena.

Nevertheless, suppose we do want to have such a complete understanding. In that case, we must understand each peculiarity of each case and the relation between the cases. Reality is relational, and the whole of existence is interrelated, including ourselves as knowers. Therefore, a complete understanding of the universe is impossible, and Whitehead acknowledges that we cannot but make abstractions (Whitehead, 1967). It is inevitable to investigate tiny pieces of reality as if they were separate entities that can be considered apart, just as gear wheels in a clock. However — and this is a task that bioethicists and philosophers can take at heart — it is crucial to refrain from thinking that these abstractions bring one closer to scientific certainty than looking at concrete phenomena would. This is reminiscent of Van Rensselaer Potter's plea for bioethics which acknowledges the limits of a scientific practice solely invested in studying mechanisms. As Whitehead says: 'beware of certitude' (Whitehead and Price, 2001). Reality, in all its concreteness, is only partially knowable.

I find the idea particularly insightful that our need for abstractions is at least partly inspired by a desire to make science workable. I am reminded about the search for genes in autism. Autism is often presented as a 'genetic' condition, probably due to its high heritability. As we have seen before, having a high heritability is not necessarily synonymous with being able to localize, on a molecular level, a stretch of atypical DNA in people diagnosed with autism. Nevertheless, it suggests that the aim of autism genetics and autism research, in general, could be finding this atypicality. Much has been written about this endeavour to assign autism as a genetic condition. One reason for this could be the exculpatory nature of genetic explanations: the firmer something is fixed in our biology, the less we can change it, or so it feels. Parents of children with challenging behaviour are, to some extent, released from a feeling of guilt as such an explanation implies that their child is not ill-behaved and, by implication, they have not failed to 'parent' correctly. The child is autistic. A genetic explanation of autism may enhance this effect even further. In any case, such explanations are an improvement to early psychogenic explanations, where a child's autism was explained by referring to the mother's behaviour. I think this is only part of the explanation of why genetic research in autism has taken such a rise in the last decades. Autism is a complex phenomenon, just like most behaviours. Furthermore, it is a developmental phenomenon, despite the insistence on it being innate and lifelong. Autistic behaviour develops over a lifetime and will evolve depending on age and context. In that respect, it is remarkable that an explanation for autism in genetic terms is so appealing. After all, what can we really know about the challenges autistic people face when we find an associated gene? However, studying actual development, especially of complex organisms such as human beings, is messy and challenging, and perhaps even out of the reach of science, given the way it is mainly practised these days. In order to truly understand autism and its development, I suggest we would need longitudinal studies spanning decades. In these studies, intricate models should be made of interactions between genes and environments, where the environment is all that an organism encounters, internally and externally. As they need to incorporate this open environment, such models are never complete: even grasping the concreteness of individual lives will always mean making abstractions. Understandably, scientists would be overwhelmed by such a project. The way scientific research is funded does not help either: scientists compete for funding that typically lasts four years and needs a definite finality: an answer to a research question. If scientists acquire funding, it is often to hire temporary junior researchers (whose contracts usually end in a PhD thesis, and this must contain tangible results to qualify for the degree).

Such results are expected to convey something generalizable about the phenomenon at hand. Searching for a genetic variant in a subset of the autistic population fits the type of research feasible in this frame. I believe this research is valuable, and I think Whitehead would agree. The 'gene for autism' is an abstraction, and it would be dangerous to neglect this. 'Autism as a genetic disorder' is only one way of seeing something already very abstract. One of our tasks as bioethicists could be to continue pointing this out to researchers and committees. After all, 'gene' is already an abstraction of the cell nucleus's messy and interconnected molecular functioning. Also, autism as a concept is an abstraction from the actual and diverse experiences of people diagnosed with it. Therein lies the danger of abstractions: they divert our attention from the concrete reality of experiences. As bioethicists serving on panels judging research proposals, our task is to make sure there is also a place for concrete case studies and experiences. These may not teach us general and abstract 'truths', but their value lies in revealing the messy relatedness and contingency of the world. The ethics appeal for the researcher in a scientific project is to be aware and question the abstractions they are making, whether they are adequate for the specific research question, and whether they are warranted. Rather than bringing us closer to certitude, abstractions may shield the peculiarities of particular cases.

A peculiar Whiteheadian idea is the fallacy of misplaced concreteness. Whitehead writes about this fallacy in *Science and the Modern World*, a more accessible book than *Process and Reality* (Whitehead, 1967). This fallacy is also known as reification. It is constructing an abstract entity as a concrete, physical thing. Reification is a term used in reference to psychiatric disorders or neurodevelopmental conditions. These are often diagnosed using behavioural descriptions. For example, the diagnosis of Attention Deficit Hyperactivity Disorder (ADHD) is given to a child based on criteria from a diagnostic manual. Today this is most often the fifth edition of the Diagnostic and Statistical Manual of Mental Disorders or DSM-5 (American Psychiatric Association, 2013). These manuals usually describe behavioural characteristics, and the DSM remains relatively agnostic as to what causes this behaviour (for example, a 'gene', a 'brain malfunction'). A diagnosis of ADHD would usually imply assessing whether someone is sufficiently inattentive and hyperactive. Hence, the diagnosis of ADHD is an abstraction, a description of various similar behaviours that can be gathered under that term. However, as Trudy Dehue rightly argues in *Betere Mensen*, the diagnosis of ADHD also functions as an explanation. A child is inattentive because they 'have' ADHD (Dehue, 2014). The behavioural diagnosis becomes tied up with a biological (neurological, genetic, etc.) explanation, even if there was never any brain scan or genetic test. This collapsing of an abstract concept into a perceived essence is reification.

That does not necessarily mean that reification is automatically a bad thing. Suppose we assume that the diagnostic criteria in the DSM are sufficiently reliable, and clinicians would come to the same conclusion when presented with similar cases. In that case, we can assume that there 'is' something to the idea that ADHD is not merely a behaviour but also a specific identity. Furthermore, there are benefits to being identified as belonging to a group of recognizable people with similar minds and shared experiences. Some interventions have proven to help with challenging symptoms. True, we do not need to reify the idea of a specific diagnosis for that. However, conceptualizing recognizable phenomena such as ADHD and autism as phenomena that can be short-circuited to biological things such as brains and genes does normative work. In my empirical work with adults with a recent diagnosis of autism, the idea of having a different brain sometimes helps self-acceptance. It makes autism as an identity real. The often-held idea that autism and ADHD are not 'real' disorders, and are made up, is experienced as harmful by many who have these diagnoses (Hens and Langenberg, 2018).

At the same time, reification and essentializing certain phenomena also have their drawbacks. Because of the idea that specific diagnoses are biological, they are often seen as static and lifelong. For some people, this may lead to despair. It may lead to overtly medicalizing certain types of behaviour. Furthermore, it can lead to dilemmas for diagnosticians. They are often aware that little is known about the biology of diagnoses based on behaviour. Still, they know that explaining this to their clients using 'brain talk' may help self-acceptance. For the biomedical ethicist considering diagnostic labels, reification is not enough reason to reject such diagnoses. But acknowledging the complex relation between diagnosis and biology should be part of any ethical consideration. Looking at biology in a dynamic and open-ended way, influenced by and influencing the way we talk about it, may help deal with the paradox of labels.

8. Time, Culture and Creativity

Time Is of the Essence

In their work on the history and topics of bioethics, Ari Schick challenges anticipatory or speculative bioethics (Schick, 2016). Speculative bioethics is a type that considers potential future developments rather than present-day medical-ethical dilemmas. Since the advent of new genetic technologies, bioethicists have often concerned themselves with speculative technologies, with possible future technologies and techniques. A good example is the belief that geneticists will be able to create designer babies, babies with desired characteristics such as athleticism or a high IQ. As bioethicists, then, it is our task to reflect on the kind of future that we might have if this ever becomes possible. This type of bioethics is trendy, and it is no wonder that the movie GATTACA is often referenced or even shown in bioethics classes. I plead guilty. The pandemic that started in 2020 has made the question of the relevance of such speculative bioethics all the more necessary: we are confronted with a banal but devastating infectious disease. At the same time, an ethical reflection of how to deal with the myriad moral dilemmas that such a pandemic would raise is sorely needed.

Schick argues that such speculative or anticipatory ethics is not only about thinking about possible futures and about being prepared for what future technologies may bring. Such reflection about the future also shapes the present. This is the 'science fictionality' of speculative bioethics. There is an opportunity cost of thinking about futures that may never happen rather than more mundane topics such as resource allocation during pandemics. However, there is an additional problem. The example of genetic embryo editing of human embryos is a good one. Taking for granted the idea that we can make future humans smarter or

     https://doi.org/10.11647/OBP.0320.08

more athletic reinforces the way we look at organisms and traits. As I will argue in Part Three, concepts related to technological enhancement entrench a reductionist and static view of organisms. The problem is not whether technology and knowledge will ever create enhanced human beings. The problem is that we think we are, in principle, enhance-able and that this is the starting point of many ethical reflections. Still, I would argue that bioethics must be forward-looking. I agree with Van Rensselaer Potter that what is at stake is the survival of the human species and, I would add, many other species as well. Guaranteeing such a future should guide our bioethical decisions. At the same time, I contend that we must look differently at both the future and present and how they relate to the past. In what follows, I will sketch some ideas regarding time and creativity that may guide us towards actual speculative bioethics that helps build the future.

An essential aspect of Whitehead's thinking is the situatedness and historicity of events. Events, and we can take this to mean any events ranging from electrons to macroscopic events, carry in them the history of what comes before. They also allow for creating something new, something that cannot merely be reduced to what has happened before. This something new is not the result of an unlimited choice: there is a range of possibilities offered by the historical events that have occurred in its path. For Whitehead, what happened in the past is a given and cannot be changed. At the same time, what will happen in the future cannot be predicted from the past. Authors who have reflected on the implications of this direction of time are Ilya Prigogine and Isabelle Stengers. Ilya Prigogine was a Belgian chemistry professor of Russian descent who received the Nobel prize in 1977. Isabelle Stengers is a Belgian professor specializing in the philosophy of science. They worked together on several books. *Order Out of Chaos* is a well-known book, initially published in French, *La Nouvelle Alliance* (Prigogine and Stengers, 1984; Prigogine and Stengers, 1997). This new alliance is between science and humanities. *The End of Certainty* is another book by Ilya Prigogine (Prigogine and Stengers, 1997). Below, I shall give an overview of these ideas and show their relevance to bioethics.

In their work, Prigogine and Stengers firmly establish time, and the arrow of time, as constitutive to reality. Those who have studied physics in high school may remember that time is a variable in many calculations.

However, In Newtonian high school physics, time is reversible. It is one variable on an axis of space and time. This reversibility means we can calculate back trajectories and predict future events with the correct variables. A classic example is the trajectory of billiard balls. If we know certain variables, such as forces and distances, we can predict which ball will be hit and the course it will take. The idea is that we start with simplifications of situations. For example, when we first learn about gravity, energy and force and have to solve equations, the teacher asks us to forget any frictional forces present in the real world. The idea is that starting from these simple situations, we can extrapolate by adding more knowledge and variables. In the end, these simple equations are the basis of reality. Once we know all the relevant variables and have powerful computers that can calculate them, we know all there is to know. We can even predict the future and go back to what happened in the past. Reality is predictable, and the arrow of time is reversible. Although the idea of a predictable universe has been challenged by theories such as chaos theory (which is deterministic) and quantum theory (which is probabilistic), this idea of a predictable universe is deeply ingrained in how we see the world. Intuitively, from a specific view of science, the future can be pre-stated, to use Stuart Kauffman's words (Kauffman, 2016). After all, science is about certainty and universal laws. At heart, reality is deterministic. Admittedly, we do not experience time like classical physics assumes time works. Subjectively, we experience a non-reversible arrow of time. Often, it is assumed that the irreversible arrow of time, and the experience of past, present and future, is constructed by those experiencing it. It is phenomenology. Entropy, of a move towards more disorder, suggests that there is such an arrow of time. After all, it is not easy to go back from a more disordered state to an ordered state. In classical conceptions of reality, this irreversibility is not a fundamental property of nature. Instead, entropy is the degree to how much we do not know (yet). At the moment, we cannot go back from entropy to order because our scientific descriptions are not detailed enough, but there is hope they will be at some point.

Prigogine and Stengers disagree with the above characterization of time. Reality is not stable, not even in principle. It is unstable and evolving. At the same time, the arrow of time is also a creative force. It can create order out of chaos and new forms of coherence. It is true that in systems in equilibrium, physics seems to be governed by deterministic laws. However, this is the exception: the vast majority of reality is governed by fundamental uncertainty. Should we mourn the fact that chaos reigns? Perhaps not. It is precisely in these systems at the edge of chaos that there is freedom. New things happen. The arrow of time allows for creation. In this way, it is not the case that we are doomed to end up in a completely disordered world. Far from equilibrium, systems will try to function, to maintain themselves, and they 'choose' one of the possible ways to do so. Near chaos, there is self-organization. The resulting organization is not deterministic. It results from the creativity of the universe: things could have ended up differently. Reality bifurcates, takes a specific path, and the others are forever lost. That is the arrow of time.

Does this mean that we cannot say anything fundamental about the universe? Yes, but we should let go of the idea that the billiard model of reality is the right one. We have to use probabilistic terms to describe what happens in dynamic systems. In more simple words, this all means that the future is not a given. It is a construction. If we introduce probabilities, we also introduce chance. We cannot pre-state what will happen. The way we experience time, as irreversible, becomes the basic structure of reality. Reality is about choice, newness, and emergence, and, I would say, about the opportunities chance encounters give us. As in this worldview, creativity is omnipresent. Prigogine and Stengers advocate for a 'nouvelle alliance' of the natural sciences and the humanities (Prigogine and Stengers, 1984). We can no longer consider science as the realm of discovering eternal laws. Both natural sciences and humanities deal with reality, albeit a creative, undetermined reality. I shall come back to this idea later on in the book.

At this point, the reader probably wonders what the point is of including these paragraphs on time and reality in a book about bioethics. At the end of the book, I hope to have clarified that a world view that incorporates creativity, chance and indeterminacy should underly bioethics if we want the field to be relevant for creating a liveable future. Thus, naturalistic bioethics does not imply that we have to buy into a belief in eternal laws or a pre-statable universe. I admit that more work needs to be done to convey that message. For now, I want to focus on the idea of the arrow of time itself. I agree with the analysis by Ari Schick that a specific type of bioethics, one that uses speculative ideas about the future, is dangerous. Using speculation in our bioethical reflection needs to be guided by the knowledge that the future is not a given. It results from the choices we make now and the possibilities we create. The future is thus not a separate realm. It is firmly anchored in the present. Let us take the example of genome editing of human embryos. Many debates on this topic deal with whether it would ever be allowed to use embryo editing to enhance human beings. We use the example of the movie GATTACA in which such techniques have led to extensive discrimination and classism. We have our students imagine a future in which embryos can and will be edited to have higher IQs. The possibility of this future is almost always taken for granted. After all, everyone seems to accept that parents want a child with a high IQ. After using GATTACA and similar scenarios myself when teaching bioethics, I realize that such examples may be misguided, even dangerous. Based on my empirical research with couples in a fertility trajectory, I am less convinced of the idea that parents desire to have high-IQ children, especially when this involves reproductive technologies (Hens *et al.*, 2019). I believe that most prospective parents' wishes are far more mundane. If reproducing the natural way was possible, most people would prefer that to IVF, even if doing IVF means controlling some characteristics of the child. At the same time, I agree with Schick that stating this as a highly probable future also changes the discussion we have right now. It means turning the arrow of time backwards. We are now debating what policies should be in place to mitigate or prevent this potential future with superhumans whose genomes will be edited. We forget that the future is what we create now. Rather than thinking about the effects of possible future technologies, following the arrow of time means thinking about the future we want with the options we have right now. It is about letting go of technological determinism. It means investing in techniques, biomedical and otherwise, that will help us create a liveable future.

Bioethics can help nudge the bifurcating path in the right direction. Using science fiction to explore what can go wrong with certain technologies can be helpful. What is unhelpful is that scenarios that take a specific reductionist worldview for granted have taken up so much of our headspace. With Stengers and Prigogine, we can acknowledge that we cannot say what we will have tomorrow, only what we may have tomorrow. I would advocate for bioethics of uncertainty. Even the 'as if' of specific scenarios yield too much certainty, and this certainty can take hostage of our ethical reflection. In the same vein, uncertainty is not the same as risk, although later, I will advocate for a concept of risk that is more about uncertainty than calculating possible outcomes. At the same time, we can use art and literature to imagine a possible future that we do wish to have. First, I want to investigate the aspect of creativity some more.

World-Making: Creating and Being Created

Prigogine and Stengers present a creative world. In what follows, I shall elaborate on what this can mean for bioethics using ideas from Stuart Kauffman, Ian Hacking and Karen Barad. They help us understand that creativity is never a one-way affair: creativity is about being created as much as creating. It is about world-making as much as reflecting on the consequences of world-making. Stuart Kauffman has a background in medicine and systems biology. He is specifically interested in how life originated. In his rather technical book *The Origin of Order*, Kauffman asks himself how, in a universe that is heading towards ever more entropy, something as ordered as life can occur (Kauffman, 1993). Like Stengers and Prigogine, he believes that exciting things happen on the edge of chaos. The phase transition from non-life to life is an example. Living systems, Kauffman argues, are organized complexity. Kauffman elaborates on these ideas further in the books *Humanity in a Creative Universe* (Kauffman, 2016) and *A World Beyond Physics* (Longo, Montévil and Kauffman, 2012; Kauffman, 2016, 2019). He argues that reality and life are fundamentally *un-prestatable*: the universe is emergent, a radical becoming that is not governed by physical laws that would enable us to predict the future. Besides not knowing what will happen, it is impossible to know what *can* happen. Hence, he writes, the becoming of the universe is 'not entailed'. Therefore, we must give up on the Newtonian and even Pythagorean dream of ever finding the holy grail of the foundational laws. We may very well be without foundation; Kauffman rejects reductive materialism and scientism. He suggests a kind of panpsychism that allows for a conception of 'choosing matter', a matter that is not inert but constantly becoming. At the same time, this does not mean that there are infinite possibilities. He uses the term *adjacent possible* to refer to the possible subsequent actions or next steps that life or even matter can take. After each step, new adjacent possibles are created. This is a *historical* ontology, just as Whitehead, Prigogine, and Stengers described. According to Kauffman, the creativity of the universe is also why we are free: we *co-create adjacent* possibilities. However, to be meaningful freedom, it is always viewed in terms of opportunities or possibilities. It is not boundless. Evolution is *non-ergotic*: not all options or combinations are created. Choices are being made. New uses are being found for existing things. Kauffman often illustrates this with the example of a screwdriver. If we were to ask what the function of a screwdriver is, we probably would say that screwdrivers are for unlocking screws. We may come up with many new uses if we are asked to imagine what we can do with a screwdriver. Screwdrivers can be used to open a can of paint. They can be used to kill people. You can use the back end to hammer a thumbtack in the wall. Come to think of it, that is almost the opposite of what a screwdriver was designed for. We may feel that the possibilities of what we can do with screwdrivers are limitless. At the same time, it is impossible to write any rules regarding how to come up with the subsequent possible use of a screwdriver. The potential uses of screwdrivers are not ordered lists or governed by laws. They arise based on the opportunities offered. To develop the subsequent possible use for the screwdriver, we have to be creative and use the possibilities the universe has to offer.

Screwdrivers may be very mundane things. However, the evolution of life is full of such examples. Think about swim bladders. These organs in fish are homologous to lungs, and it is hypothesized that they acquired, through evolution, a new use for fish that breath through gills. Swim bladders help these fish float in water without having to move. The use of the swim bladder for buoyancy is an example of Kauffman's adjacent possible: it began when the organ was not strictly needed anymore for oxygen supply. Life's evolution is full of these examples of how things with a specific function evolved to another function, depending on circumstances. The constraints that are met enable new possibilities. In the same way, beings and matter are the constraints and possibilities of each other. We create each other's world and are being made by others. Suppose we accept, with Kauffman, that we live in a un-prestatable universe, where final laws can only paint a partial picture. In this universe we cannot know what will happen, but we also cannot know what can happen. In that case, creativity and metaphors can play a pivotal role besides reason. Like Stengers and Prigogine, Stuart Kauffman argues sternly against the idea of 'two cultures': metaphors can show us new possibilities, just as art and literature.

The reader may wonder how these ideas are relevant to bioethics. The ideas sketched above may feel too foreign, too weird, and maybe even too crazy for some. Some readers may intuitively reject the idea of selective electrons and creative universes. I believe they provide an ontology for what has been argued by philosopher of science Ian Hacking. With Hacking, we can leave the quantum and the cosmological level and zoom back to eye level. Ian Hacking describes how words and categories shape realities and vice versa. He calls this dynamic nominalism (Hacking, 1996, 2001, 2009, 2010). Using autism as an example, Hacking demonstrates how the way we demarcate boundaries between kinds of people creates new ways of being for these people and unavoidably changes the way people are. On an individual level, this means that a diagnosis of autism in an adult person changes how they view their past and future. On a collective level, experiences of autistic people, such as hypersensitivity to sounds or smells, may become part of the diagnosis. Experiences of challenges become interpreted as part of autism. A child diagnosed will not merely be described by a specific word, autism. The child's future and possible paths will be thoroughly influenced by the diagnosis, to the extent that we may say that the child will become a different person depending on whether the child receives a diagnosis or not. Diagnosticians and child psychiatrists are well aware of this fact, and overall, they approach diagnosis with due care.

In many cases, it is argued that the adult or child in question will benefit from a diagnosis: adequate services will be put in place, and the diagnosis will help. There may also be negative consequences: being diagnosed means that people may view you in a certain way, that specific options will be foreclosed, and others will become available. The point is that we cannot be sure what the impact of the diagnosis will be. However, the fact that a diagnosis changes someone's world is not in itself a reason why a diagnosis may be harmful. With Hacking and Kauffman, I would say a reflection on diagnoses should first acknowledge that diagnoses are not merely descriptions of phenomena or people. They are world-making. Not diagnosing will create a different world than diagnosing. As bioethicists, we should not simply reflect on the consequences of scientific facts but on the creation of these facts themselves. I have discussed this in more depth in a previous book, *Towards an Ethics of Autism* (Hens, 2021).

Ian Hacking investigates the relationship between words and things (Hacking, 2004). He is part of a long tradition of philosophers who try to understand what representation means and if representation is an adequate paradigm to characterize the relation between words and things. Dynamic nominalism is the first step in bridging the gap between words and things. As a literature student in the nineties, I was steeped in poststructuralist thinking. We took it for granted that words shape things and that things in themselves and essences are somehow unattainable for human beings, immersed as we are in the Symbolic order. Nowadays, even the staunchest representationalist would, I think, argue that the link between words and things is not as simple as a one-on-one mapping. Nevertheless, our obsession with words has caused us to neglect things and matter. As bioethicists, we deal with living and non-living things like technology. The pandemic has made it all the more relevant to reflect on our intimate relationship with the physical world. In the last two decades, some philosophers have returned to thinking about *matter*, about material phenomena. One such line of thought is new materialism. I will briefly outline the ideas of new materialist thinker Karen Barad because she describes an ethico-onto-epistemology, a vision in which ethics, epistemology, and ontology are deeply entangled. Barad's book *Meeting the Universe Halfway* is a phenomenal work, which is impossible to summarise in a few paragraphs (Barad, 2007). I shall try anyway.

Barad begins her book with Niels Bohr and Werner Heisenberg's respective interpretations of quantum mechanics. I will not delve too deeply into quantum mechanics here, but it boils down to this. We know the two-slit experiment of quantum mechanics demonstrates that we cannot simultaneously measure the momentum and locality of an electron. These two characteristics are complementary and mutually exclusive. If we measure one characteristic, we cannot determine the other. For Heisenberg, this is a question of uncertainty. The electron is disturbed by the experiment, which aims to measure its momentum and locality to such an extent that the two characteristics can never be measured together. Hence, the uncertainty is an epistemic principle: the electron may have a specific location and momentum, but we cannot know them because we have to measure them, which disturbs the electron. Simply put, if we measure the electron's position, our measuring equipment pins it down, and momentum is lost. However, for Bohr, there is more to it than a mere limitation of how we can know things. Rather than uncertainty, for Bohr, there is indeterminacy. The characteristics of location and momentum do not exist together. There is no 'real' electron with location and momentum. The electron's attributes come into existence during measurements. Here Barad departs from Bohr.

Bohr, like Heisenberg, puts human beings and their measuring equipment at the centre of his reasoning, albeit in the form of indeterminacy. However, Barad argues that humans and their language have been attributed too much power: the assumption that, on the one hand, language is dynamic and, on the other hand, matter is inert, is wrong and starts from outdated representationalism. Objects, or rather phenomena, are always in intra-action. They come into being through relations with other entities. Matter itself is what does the *mattering*. It is dynamic. Barad's is a posthumanist way of thinking: the intra-action, the relation is not only between humans and their measuring instruments and things, but it is also between everything else, even when no human is involved. Barad throws human beings from the pedestal of meaning givers: matter is agential and productive and plays a constitutive role in the world's becoming. Everything, including human beings, is an emergent phenomenon. Representationalism is wrong: there are no concepts that stand above reality. Concepts *emerge* in reality.

In other writings, I have used Barad's idea to find a new way of looking at developmental conditions such as autism. The debate about these conditions is often about their realness. However, people who would claim that 'autism is not real, it is merely a construct in language' and those who would firmly locate it in genes or a yet-to-be-defined neurological type are firmly speaking in representationalist terms. We can see autism as an absolute, historically unchanged essence that we can hunt for in science or as fictional and without an essence. Using new materialist thinking, we can think about it differently. Barad herself states that 'Quantum theory leads us out of the morass that takes absolutism and relativism to be the two only possibilities' (Barad, 2007). Using concepts such as intra-action and entanglement, we can advocate autism's realness while at the same time acknowledging the concept's dynamism and historicity. I believe investing in combatting the old representationalism regarding diagnoses and looking at these phenomena differently is an ethical endeavour. Disability scholars and crip theorists, who think about how disability interacts with experiences like race, class or gender, have already shown us that this is possible. For now, I want to focus on another part of Barad's idea relevant to bioethics. The fact that we participate in the World's becoming implies, for Barad, that we can be held accountable for what the future ends up being. At the end of *Meeting the Universe Halfway*, she writes:

> Meeting each moment, being alive to the possibilities of becoming, is an ethical call, an invitation that is written into the very matter of all being and becoming. We need to meet the universe halfway, to take responsibility for the role that we play in the World's differential becoming. (Barad, 2007, p. 396)

Ethico-onto-epistemology is the interrelatedness of ethics, being and knowing, and I contend that it is, de facto, what bioethicists practice. We think about what we should do in light of scientific practice and influence. At the same time, we are influenced by technological developments and other organisms. Ideas from new materialism can help us think through ethico-onto-epistemology and what this means for ethics. By acknowledging and advocating the use of certain words and practices, bioethicists make an 'agential cut' in reality to create new worlds. In this respect, we see this world-making as profoundly ethical. Thinkers such as Donna Haraway, Bruno Latour, Nicolas Rose, and Ian Hacking acknowledge that science does such world-making. However, it is not science and its concepts alone that engage in world-making. Practising philosophy and ethics create worlds and shuts down paths to other worlds. We must step away from the idea that we observe the world from a distance and that we describe what is and what is good from a distant archimedean vantage point.

Bioethicists are not merely engaging in the practice of making the scientific approach more ethical. Our thoughts may be but grains of sand in the desert of the world, but still, grains of sand matter. I remember discussing the idea of a 'pill for autism' during a lecture I gave at a psychology conference. Curing autism or creating a pill for autism is highly contested. Autism is a disability, a way of being that has its challenges but that is not to be eradicated. I hold this view as well. Furthermore, I agree that autism is not the kind of concept that 'curing' or 'pills' apply to. Autistic people will sometimes welcome medicinal solutions to specific problems they face, such as sensitivity to sound or sleeping problems. However, accepting treatment for issues and symptoms associated with autism is different from getting treatment for autism itself. Nevertheless, besides being a question of the ethics of genetic cleansing of certain kinds of people, the question is also one of ontology. Autism is a multidimensional and even polysemous concept. The question of what we would cure if there were such a pill is unresolvable. As I have argued elsewhere, this is different from saying that autism does not exist. Autism exists: it is a common language, a way of looking at oneself, a shared experience related to—but not mapped one-on-one with—biological function. However, this shared experience cannot be reduced to something like neurology, a gene, or a hormone susceptible to therapeutic intervention. Different neurologies or genes may yield the same shared experience, and other experiences may be linked to one neurology. At this conference, someone asked me the following question: 'What if there was a pill for autism? Do you think autistic people want to take it?' I started to answer that I think we make a category mistake if we apply 'pill' or 'cure' to autism. However, the person who asked the question, very well-versed in the complexity of the concept of autism, persisted. They said, 'but imagine, philosophically, that we could do this, what would autistic people say?' We did not have time to discuss this further. After my talk, I thought about it some more and concluded that I would even object to the use of 'autism' as a phenomenon that can be cured, even in a philosophical thought experiment. There is something completely different about a fictional example such as curing autism and a fictional example such as brains in a vat or a violinist that needs to be provided with blood from an attached living person for nine months. There is also a difference with potentially realistic scenarios about cures for specific challenges associated with autism, such as difficulties sleeping or hypersensitivity to sound. Using 'a cure for autism' as an example in a thought experiment and asking people to imagine that autism is a phenomenon that can be cured implies that we are turning an ontological issue into an ethical one. We are suggesting that the ontological issue is something irrelevant. We are also contributing to the persistence of a world in which people mistakenly believe in the curability of autism. Such world-making or world-maintaining, for that matter, is ethically relevant. The same goes for thought experiments of the type 'what if we could genetically modify embryos to be smarter?' In the latter case, we persist with the idea that, in principle, more intelligent is better or that we even know what 'smart' means. Category mistakes, even intentional ones in a fictional thought experiment, are not harmless. We should be aware of the worlds we make, not only because of the conclusions we may draw but also through the words we use and the ideas we keep alive.

9. Symbiosis and Interdependency

In the previous paragraphs, I have described the dynamics of matter, of the relationality of things as phenomena. The posthuman ontology of new materialism and the Whiteheadian tradition of process philosophy seems suitable for ethics that seeks to examine and advocate our world's flourishing and sustenance. Many bioethicists try to grasp the impact of technologies, how they affect decisions, and whether they should be welcomed or forbidden. If new materialist thinkers have a point, we may want to question technologies more fundamentally than seeing them as tools humans can misuse. There is still much leeway for cooperation between bioethicists and Science and Technology Studies scholars, who have thought about the agency of technologies in depth. However, the main aim of this book is to think about bioethics as the ethics of life. In this last chapter of Part Two, I want to go back to life and the question of how we must conceive of life and our relationship with all types of life. Indeed, although it may be impossible for human beings and bioethics not to be primarily focused on matters that concern humans, I think if we take posthumanism seriously, we must also acknowledge our entanglement with other forms of life. Furthermore, we must spread our net across domains and kingdoms, including fungi and microorganisms. Recent authors, biologists and anthropologists have explored the mushroom as a world builder. Anthropologist Anna Lowenhaupt Tsing describes how the Matsutake mushroom, a delicacy in Japan, shapes the worlds of people trying to make a living across the globe in her brilliant book *The Mushroom at the End of the World* (Tsing, 2015). Merlin Sheldrake described the secret life of fungi in his *Entangled Life* (Sheldrake, 2021). He points out that fungi have influenced the existence of plant and animal life and human life in general across history. Some scholars argue that the hallucinogenic properties may have opened up undiscovered roads of imagination in early humans.

 https://doi.org/10.11647/OBP.0320.09

Through the invention of penicillin, fungi may even have altered the course of the world's history, and, studies suggest, they may help fight against environmental pollution. Fungi are a testament to how life, as we know it, may have been the result of chance encounters with other living beings, maybe as much as it is the result of gene selection for fitness. Insights about how our lives are entangled with fungi may have philosophical repercussions for ontology and epistemology. Rather than asking ourselves how we as human beings are unique, which we have been doing for over twenty centuries, we may start to ask ourselves how we are entangled with other beings.

In the first part of this book, I have described how new findings in molecular biology have challenged the reductionist view that sees organisms as mere mechanisms, the result of programs written in our genes. Epigenetics and similar findings have demonstrated that a more developmental view of organisms, constantly interacting with their environment, building and being built by their milieu, is closer to the truth. Recent findings in microbiology show us that the story is even more complex. Besides their entanglement with the physical and cultural environment, humans are also entangled with the billions of microorganisms that live in the gut and elsewhere in the body. Just as epigenetics can challenge a gene-centric view of life, the gut microbiome challenges the brain-centric view of human cognition. The impact of the gut microbiome on well-being and even on the mental state is believed to be so huge that the gut is sometimes called 'the second brain'. Compared with the enormous amount of bioethics literature written about genes and the growing corpus written on epigenetics, bioethicists have paid relatively little attention to the ethical questions surrounding research on and clinical applications of the gut microbiome. Many such questions require further investigation. They include questions about privacy, the phenotypical personal information gathered from our microbiome, safety issues related to faecal transplants, and ethical questions related to the biobanking of such material (Rhodes, 2016). Fundamental questions relate to personal identity: what is our identity, if who we are is defined by bacteria in our gut (Ma *et al.*, 2018)? In this respect, Yonghui Ma and colleagues write: 'We might need to reconceptualize the human body as an ecosystem and the human being as a superorganism, rather than being a single individual' (Ma *et al.*, 2018). I believe one of the significant challenges for bioethics and science in the twenty-first century is reconceptualizing our relationship with the microbial world. Ethical questions surrounding the gut-brain microbiome, inquiries related to antibiotic resistance, the harmful effects on beneficial bacteria of necessary hygiene measures during a pandemic, and the complex relationship we have with them are awaiting scrutinous investigation. Such reflection should include a proper analysis of our relationship with the world on a macro and micro scale. But I leave this thought for another time. Here, I want to briefly sketch the ideas of a brilliant thinker who has influenced how we look at the earth and our place within it. This thinker is microbiologist Lynn Margulis.

Margulis challenges the standard neo-Darwinist view on organisms in the twentieth century. For her, neo-Darwinism 'took the life out of biology' (Margulis, 2008). Genes do as described, but a narrow focus on genes suggests a mechanistic and reductive view on life. Margulis has described life by tracing it back to its origins and championed the idea of the cell as the primary unit of life. Nevertheless, the nucleated cell as we know it in animals, plants and fungi only developed 1.5 billion years after the first forms of life appeared on the earth. Margulis fights the idea that nothing much of interest happened before that period. Instead, she states in the documentary *Symbiotic Earth: How Lynn Margulis Rocked the Boat and Started a Scientific Revolution*:[1] 'everything happened'. Blue-green algae, their descendants still with us today, started to give up oxygen. Their waste product created an atmosphere in which later life could thrive. Margulis wrote in 1967 that the nucleated cell originated through symbiotic mergers of bacteria. This idea was not new, but she positioned it firmly as crucial in life's history. With the advent of DNA sequencing techniques, her thoughts were proven through experiments: chloroplasts and mitochondria can now be traced back to bacteria. Not only is our health and functioning dependent on microbes in our gut and cells — cells being the basic units of life — but it is also the result of bacterial mergers. For Margulis, such symbiosis between different species plays a vital role in speciation. From the moment living cells appeared on earth, organisms worked together to the extent that they merged. Such 'cooperation' is an essential aspect of speciation, just as

---

1   https://vimeo.com/ondemand/symbioticearthhv

much as the idea of survival of the fittest. It gives an alternative to the tale of a cruel world in which only the strongest survive. It may also influence how we look at cells and the nucleus. We may have looked at the cytoplasm too much as the cell's periphery and considered the nucleus too much as the core thing, the heart of the cell. However, realizing that the cytoplasm contains organelles that were, in ancient history, separate beings can function as a wake-up call that there is yet much to discover about life and the cell. It has always struck me as weird, for example, that the things that do the work in the cell, proteins, have received far less attention from ethicists than genes. The explanation is probably because proteins are seen as the 'result' of mechanisms that start with the genes. They are the 'product'. However, proteins are complex three-dimensional structures that actively shape and influence a cell's workings. They are linked with the environment and contain more information about the organism's phenotype than its genes.

Furthermore, let us consider the mitochondria. Mitochondrial DNA in human beings contains 37 genes, far fewer than nuclear DNA, but they have drawn the attention of bioethicists. They are of bacterial origin and play an essential role in cell metabolism. Mutations in mitochondrial DNA can lead to diseases with different levels of severity. In 2014, I was assigned a small project as a postdoctoral researcher on the ethics of a new *in vitro* technique that would help women at risk of transferring a mitochondrial disease to potential children using a nuclear transfer technique. A donor's zygote, a fertilized oocyte, is enucleated. The nucleus of an oocyte of the prospective mother is also removed and put into the zygote. The resulting zygote had the nuclear DNA of the prospective parent, who will typically also give birth to the child, but the cytoplasm with the non-affected mitochondrial DNA of the donor.

Since 2015, children have been born that were conceived with this technique. I interviewed several clinicians and researchers with opinions on the matter (Hens, Dondorp and de Wert, 2015). What struck me was that most of the professionals in favour of the technique praised the fact that this would allow women to have a child that was their own genetically, but the child would be free from mitochondrial disease. These professionals rejected the name by which the technique had become known in popular media as 'three-parent baby'. There were only two parents. The mitochondria were donated, but these organelles play no role in genetic relatedness, so it was said. They are merely the energy factories of the cell. However, in terms of the space it takes, the nucleus is only a tiny part of the cell. In this view, the contribution of the cytoplasm donor is significant. The rationale that what is vital for relatedness between parents and their children is passing on one's nuclear DNA is, while understandable, somewhat short-sighted. We may wonder whether such relatedness is so essential that one would prefer to undergo an experimental technique to pass nuclear DNA on to one's offspring. It would be possible to use the entire oocyte of a donor, a tried and far more straightforward technique. This question puzzled me and puzzles me still. Indeed mitochondrial DNA's effect on the child's health is so significant that as much as possible is done to prevent it from being passed onto the child. Suppose what is at stake is the identity-affecting aspect of nuclear DNA. In that case, whether or not one has a mitochondrial disease seems pretty identity-affecting. Maybe the number of genes in mitochondrial DNA or, as a doctor once told me, the fact that it is thought to be only transferred by women causes it to be seen as less important. Maybe the desire to pass on nuclear DNA to one's children is not solely about the identity features of the child but about having children that are like you as much as possible. However, even in the case of natural conception, this is not guaranteed. Moreover, we can question whether the desire to have children resemble oneself is important enough in the grand scheme of things to research and implement expensive procedures. We may have been wrong all along when taking the relative importance of nuclear DNA for granted in discussions about reproductive techniques. Reassessing the role of the cytoplasm and of everything that goes on in the cell that is not nuclear DNA will, I think, shed new light on these debates. Thinking with Lynn Margulis may help to refocus the ethical questions themselves.

In this part, I suggested how a view on life consistent with a process ontology is relevant for bioethics. Using ideas from Whitehead, Stengers, Prigogine, Barad and Margulis, I described an ontology in which historicity and development are fundamental: our history is incorporated into who we are. Besides this historicity, this ontology is also one of indeterminacy and unpredictability. We cannot predict future events with certainty. They are as much the results of choices and opportunities as they are the result of deterministic laws. It is precisely that unpredictability that suggests an element of creativity in choosing future paths. Moreover, choices and opportunities are shaped by relations and by chance encounters with other organisms and things. In the spirit of Lynn Margulis, life, as we know it, may in itself be the result of such chance encounters. As human beings, we may have to imagine ourselves again as beings among other beings beyond anthropocentric humanism. As situated beings, this means giving up the idea that absolute truth is there to find if we try hard enough. This is true as much for ethics as it is for science. However, this does not mean we have to resort to relativism. Instead, it means committing to both epistemic and ethical humility and acknowledging that to be able to understand things, we must investigate experiences and situated knowledge. What this means will be the subject of Part Three.

In the previous paragraphs, I have mainly relayed and challenged ideas from Global North thinkers who view human beings as atomistic individuals at the top of either creation or the end-point of evolution. While writing this book, I became increasingly aware that this is only one possible approach amongst many others that have been forgotten or deliberately put away as folklore rather than philosophy. Both atomistic ideas of humankind and their relation to the environment and recent thinkers that react against that are but one thread in the history of philosophy. The same goes for current endeavours that try to think beyond existing dualisms of nature-nurture, genes-environment, and man-woman. Such 'thinking beyond' already assumes a dualistic 'before' that we should transcend. In many different cultures, these dualisms never were so crucial in the first place. For example, Nigerian feminist scholar Oyèrónkẹ́ Oyěwùmí gives the example of the Yorùbá society, where concepts such as 'woman' and 'gender' did not play a fundamental structural role (Oyěwùmí, 1997). By focussing on the Western story as the only genuinely 'philosophical' story of philosophy, we have missed crucial opportunities to think differently. I cannot do justice to the many rich ways of thinking about the relationship between humans and their environment. I think it is not my place to interpret and use indigenous thinking, as I still have so much learning to do in that respect. I want to end this chapter with a quote from *How It Is—the Native American Philosophy of V.F. Cordova*. The words speak for themselves but please also read the entire book.

I exist only in and as a context. I am what the context has created. I did not burst full bloom into the world. I confront. I do not have a 'hidden', 'inner' or 'true' self that lies waiting for my discovery. I have been created by an experience, and I am recreated — over and over again — by each new experience (Cordova, 2007).

PART THREE: EXPERIENCE

In which I investigate concepts of disease and the importance of experience

---

Life is Experience

– Georges Canguilhem (Canguilhem, 2008)

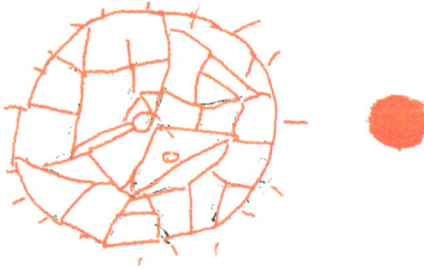

re-Visioning Red Night Light.

How to perceive microbial agents inside the eye itself (entoptic) without technological or phytochemical means?

Sketch by Bartaku, June 2021[1]

---

1   Series of experiments for enhanced microtuning, awakening and practicing sensorial empathies, in this case using entoptic vision: learning to see pathogenic microbes in the sapiens bloodstream without a microscope. Inspired by Giraldo Herrera, *Microbes and other Shamanic Beings* (Cham: Palgrave Macmillan, 2018).

In Part One, I argued that it is part of the task of the bioethicist to team up with philosophers of science and question scientific concepts and assumptions that structure both scientific and bioethical thinking. I used the dichotomy between nature and nurture and the reductionist vision of life as programmed in genes as examples of such assumptions. I suggested a developmental way of looking at organisms, including human beings. Such a dynamic and developmental approach also sheds new light on old discussions surrounding the ethics of genetics. In Part Two, I sketched an ontology for the bioethics of the twenty-first century. Imminent catastrophes, such as climate change, and ongoing ones, such as the pandemic, force us to rethink humanity's position regarding the environment. A purely anthropocentric approach is insufficient in situations where humankind's survival depends on forces beyond our control. That does not mean that defeatism is all that is left. A process ontology firmly positions us with other organisms and things but also suggests that there is room for creativity.

Creativity is at the heart of the universe. Human beings are no longer the masters of a world they can manipulate to shape the future. Neither are they merely victims of forces beyond their control. Human beings can work with the world to create a liveable future. Bioethics that inscribes itself in such a process account comes close to what Potter imagined in his first book *Bioethics, a Bridge to the Future* (Potter, 1971). I suggest that endorsing process ontology, because it asserts the situatedness of knowledge, implies endorsing the importance of experiences, a step Potter does not explicitly take. At the same time, bioethics has become firmly associated with biomedical ethics and clinical practice. This association presupposes that bioethics is also an ethics of the personal choices patients and clinicians make in specific cases. In Part Three, we discuss diseases and disabilities to pave the way for an approach that imagines the private sphere of medical ethics and the public sphere of environmental ethics together, a step we shall take in Part Four.

10. Medical Ethics and Environmental Ethics

In his first book, Van Rensselaer Potter imagined bioethics as a biology-based discipline that would help the survival of humanity. In his 1988 book, *Global Bioethics*, he concedes that in the years since writing *Bioethics, Bridge to the Future*, the term bioethics has come to mean something different (Potter, 1971; Potter, 1988). Indeed, in the seventies and eighties, bioethics was, he explains, being developed as an outgrowth of medical ethics at Georgetown University and the Hastings Institute. Indeed, until today, bioethics is still associated primarily with questions surrounding the ethics of reproduction, euthanasia, advance directives, informed consent, and privacy issues related to genetic research and the like. Environmental ethics is not automatically associated with bioethics, although many bioethics syllabi have an entry on environmental ethics. However, questions about biotechnology and animals for research already call for an interaction between medical ethics and environmental ethics.

Bioethics is a discipline that primarily studies practices and developments in the biomedical field. The type of bioethics that Potter envisaged in his 1971 book never made it to the mainstream. He writes:

> Medical bioethics and ecological bioethics are non-overlapping in the sense that medical bioethics is chiefly concerned with short-term views: the options open to individuals and their physicians in their attempts to prolong life through the use of organ transplants, artificial organs, experimental chemotherapy, and all the newer developments in the field of medicine. Ecological bioethics clearly has a long-term view that is concerned with what we must do to preserve the ecosystem in a form that is compatible with the continued existence of the human species. (Potter, 1988).

 https://doi.org/10.11647/OBP.0320.10

In both books, Potter believes the primary goal of bioethics must be the survival of humankind. Such survival means, for him, that there should be population control. Indeed, Potter, in his two books, considered the question of overpopulation as maybe the most pressing issue of his (ecological) ethics. This idea seems far removed from medical ethics, specifically its subdiscipline, reproductive ethics. In reproductive ethics, the right of people to reproduce is seldomly questioned. Perhaps we have been too myopic in avoiding such questions. When teaching students about reproductive ethics, I sometimes ask them about the ethical issues related to new reproductive technologies. When I have them reflect on topics such as gene editing of human embryos, their standard answers relate to designer babies or the right of parents to choose their type of child. Some students, particularly from the biology curriculum, would, from time to time, mention the question of overpopulation: they would question the idea that we should invest in technologies that would create even more people. Bioethicists should not shy away from difficult questions regarding the assumptions we take for granted, such as the right of people to reproduce and have as many children as they want. At the same time, we must also consider the plight of those who cannot reproduce naturally but wish to have children. Potter is naïve in his assumption that fighting overpopulation is the primary way to solve the world's problems. To his credit, he does not suggest population control should be forced upon people: It should be accomplished through education around birth control, provision of contraception, fighting poverty, and ensuring women receive a good standard of education after the age of 11. At the same time, he sometimes is ableist when discussing abortion and the management of pre-term newborns. I shall come back to that later.

Nevertheless, making more people, an aim of reproductive medicine, is an excellent example of how medical bioethics and environmental ethics sometimes speak different languages. Principles such as reproductive autonomy or even procreative beneficence and references to individual rights and responsibilities seem incompatible with global goals. However, back in 1988, Potter acknowledged that medical and environmental issues should not be considered separately: 'The time has come to recognize that we can no longer examine medical options without considering ecological science and the larger problems of society on a global scale' (1988, Global Bioethics) (Potter, 1988). Since the beginning of 2020, humanity has faced a global challenge in the form of a pandemic. The quote from Potter seems visionary. That health and environment are intrinsically linked seems a truism, but one that we may have neglected. The origins of pandemics have been linked with biodiversity loss (Jones *et al.*, 2008; Dobson *et al.*, 2020). Infectious respiratory diseases are probably worse for those suffering from respiratory problems due to pollution (Pozzer *et al.*, 2020). In his book *Wounded Planet*, Henk ten Have also recognizes the urgency of Potter's legacy, as health and environment can no longer be seen as separate spheres:

> Climate change, toxic waste, air pollution, ozone depletion, extreme weather events, and loss of biodiversity have had significant impacts on health and healthcare. Deforestation and destruction of habitat are associated with the emergence of new viral diseases such as Ebola or Zika. Focusing on care, treatment, or vaccination of individual patients can thus not be disconnected from the wider environmental context in the management of epidemics. (ten Have, 2019, p. 2)

Furthermore, the sphere of the biomedical is no longer completely private in a pandemic: who gets access to vaccines and treatment is a question of global justice. My ambition is not to solve the seeming incompatibility of medical ethics, public health, and environmental justice. The balancing act of thinking of the two together is at the heart of what it means to practice bioethics. In what follows, I shall explore what this could imply using some of the ideas discussed in Parts One and Two. I shall first revisit the philosophical discussion about concepts of disease and the enhancement debate, which has been at the core of many bioethics discussions. I shall briefly describe the ideas of Georges Canguilhem as a philosopher who fits the idea of a situated and developmental approach to medicine. With Canguilhem, I will explore the importance of standpoints and individual experiences. In Part Four, I suggest an approach to bioethics that covers both private relations and public responsibilities.

11. Diseases, Disorders, Disabilities, and Norms

> The concept is thus the friend of all those seeking radical social change, who seek new events and new alignments of forces.
>
> – Elizabeth Grosz (Grosz, 2011, p. 80)

Diseases: What They Are and Why It Matters

After the first wave of the COVID-19 pandemic in 2020, many people reported long-lasting fatigue, concentration problems, pain in the chest and muscles, and loss of smell and taste. A significant percentage of people who had experienced what was then called 'mild' symptoms of COVID-19, meaning that they had not been hospitalized, now suffer from long COVID-19 to the extent that some of them are unable to work. Having experienced this myself, I realised first-hand the implications of thinking about a phenomenon as a 'real' disease. Indeed, at the beginning of the pandemic, many professionals were sceptical about the phenomenon. It was often thought to be 'all in one's head' due to lockdown depression or a frail personality. The World Health Organization acknowledges that long COVID-19 is a 'real' phenomenon (*The Lancet*, 2020). This acknowledgement has significant consequences. It means that long COVID-19 has become an object of scientific research. Public health authorities acknowledge it as a valid reason for sick leave or reimbursement. For the patients themselves, it means credibility. They do not have an imaginary disease. At the same time, people with other similar symptoms, such as chronic fatigue syndrome, which may have been caused by a viral infection that is no longer detectable, still struggle for an acknowledgement.

© 2022 Kristien Hens, CC BY-NC-ND 4.0   https://doi.org/10.11647/OBP.0320.11

These examples demonstrate that there is much at stake: whether something is considered a genuine disease or not has profound implications. On the one hand, symptoms that are thought to be related to 'real' diseases are taken seriously by the medical profession and the public. On the other hand, if we are too eager to call a phenomenon a 'disease', this can lead to excess medicalization. Specifically, this danger is real when we think about developmental and mental phenomena. Is being very hyperactive or inattentive a sign of 'the disease' ADHD? If we answer this question with a yes, we will probably be more eager to suggest medication. On the flip side of medicalization, there is also the ethical debate on enhancement. If we decide that a specific phenomenon is not a disease but is part of what we consider normal health, intervening to ameliorate that phenomenon is considered enhancement. As I shall discuss later in this chapter, for many, whether something is an enhancement or a treatment has normative implications if we consider the acceptability of specific technologies and procedures.

Moreover, if we consider something a disease, the phenomenon will more readily be regarded as a valid object of clinical research into its causes, such as genes. This, in turn, leads to new ethical questions as to whether we should 'know' this about children even before they are born and whether foetuses or embryos with genes for inattention are targets for selection or even embryo editing. At the same time, although the question about the delineation between health and disease carries such normative weight, there is no strict line to be drawn. What is health, and what is a disease? Is someone with high blood pressure, but without other symptoms, ill? Do we need 'proof' to consider a phenomenon a disease, as in the case of long COVID-19? In an age where preventive medicine has taken flight, this question becomes all the more pertinent, as biomarkers and symptoms will no longer be straightforwardly linked. Although there is a rich corpus of philosophical literature on concepts of health, disease and disability, conceptual reflection on what makes a particular variant an actual disease is often absent in much bioethics literature. Still, engagement with this writing is necessary for bioethicists. First, reflecting on health and disease reveals a fundamentally normative component about what we consider a disease: naming something a disease entails that this is something to be avoided or cured. Second, biological notions play a normative role in diagnosing and aetiology (causation) of disease. As becomes apparent when looking at phenomena such as depression or chronic disease, naming a specific biological 'cause' of a disease, such as a gene or a pathogen, can be liberating: it relieves patients of responsibility and blame. It may, however, also lead to stigmatisation (Phelan, 2005; Kvaale, Haslam and Gottdiener, 2013).

What are diseases? Is it possible to define once and for all criteria that would delineate diseases from non-diseases? Philosophers have tried; there is a whole entry in the *Stanford Encyclopaedia of Philosophy* on the debate (Murphy, 2021). Often in these discussions, two different views are juxtaposed (Stegenga, 2018). One is the naturalist view, in which it is assumed that there are some natural qualities that phenomena must have to qualify as 'disease'. This apparently makes sense, given the intrinsic link between 'disease' and (biomedical) science. Think about the example of long COVID-19 that I have used. For many, long COVID-19 is at least a candidate to be considered a 'real disease' if it is associated with a specific infection detected in the body. Nevertheless, this is problematic in different aspects. First, there is the possibility of a false negative, the chance that the test gave a negative result but there was still a COVID-19 infection. It is possible that a specific patient's complaints are due to a previous COVID-19 infection but that the patient no longer has antibodies. Hence, they cannot deliver proof that they are suffering from long COVID-19. Second, the line between symptoms and diseases proper is also hard to draw. With regard to long COVID-19, we do not know if this is different from other post-viral reactions, nor to what extent it matters. The symptoms in themselves seem debilitating enough to warrant further investigation. Disease causes or 'primal events' such as a viral infection may shed some light on treating the long-term consequences. At the same time, much work could be done to help patients with similar symptoms regardless of their cause.

Christopher Boorse is perhaps the most known and influential proponent of the naturalist approach to disease. For Boorse, we can lay down reference classes of organisms' functioning based on age and sex (Boorse, 1977, 1997). Species-typical functioning concerns itself with normal bodily function—reproduction as an example—and defines 'normal' in relation to other organisms in the same reference class based on age and sex. Health means having an average functional ability in the species-typical functioning. A disease is an internal state impairing health. An organism or an organ is diseased if the organism is no longer functioning at that typical level. This is a biostatistical approach to health and disease: disease implies deviance from the statistical mean, and typical (and healthy) organs or organisms function at the mean of a bell curve. Many have argued that such a naturalist approach is insufficient and potentially harmful. This may be especially true for what we consider mental diseases. First, it may very well be impossible to find genuinely universal species-typical functioning of human beings. Species-typical functioning, especially related to cognitive or behavioural phenomena, is also related to cultural expectations. For example, in diagnostic tools for autism developed in the Global North, atypical eye contact is considered part of the autistic phenotype. However, looking adults in the eye may be abnormal and even pathological behaviour in some cultures but may be expected and even polite in other cultures. Extreme tallness and homosexuality are also phenomena that may not be considered part of 'species-typical functioning'. At the same time, they are certainly not diseases. Especially in the case of sexual orientation, the species-typical approach may even be dangerous, as it can lead to unwarranted pathologizing. True, Christopher Boorse himself actively tried to counter these critiques by stating that it is not necessary for a disease to always be considered bad per se (Boorse, 1975). Nevertheless, I doubt it is possible to strip disease of its normative connotation. In fact, by saying that something is a disease, this is not a harmless description but is an implication and assumption that something is bad to have and may even be contributing to the making of disease. I shall come back to this later.

Other philosophers of medicine take a normativist approach to disease judgements. This is often assumed to mean that it is a disease if it is an undesirable or disvalued state for an individual or a society. For example, Rachel Cooper, a proponent of the normativist approach to concepts of disease, states that:

> By 'disease' we aim to pick out a variety of conditions that through being painful, disfiguring or disabling are of interest to us as people. No biological account of disease can be provided because this class of conditions is by its nature anthropocentric and corresponds to no natural class of conditions in the world (Cooper, 2002).

Hence, we cannot separate what we judge as a disease from human values. The negative evaluation of a medical or bodily condition makes it a disease. That does not mean that such evaluation should be taken for granted. Human values can be wrong, as in the case of thinking that homosexuality is a disease. People who believe homosexuality is a disease are misguided, perhaps malevolent. However, we should ask if just a negative evaluation of something is enough to qualify it as a disease. Disease, linked with medicine and biology, also evokes the idea of pathology, something happening in our bodies or minds. Therefore, some authors have suggested hybridist conceptions of disease. For example, in his book *Medical Nihilism*, Jacob Stegenga argues for a hybridist solution in which naturalism and normativism are jointly sufficient but mutually exclusive (Stegenga, 2018). A workable disease concept should include both function and value.

Normative conceptions of disease are attractive. They make clear that we cannot separate disease from its negative connotation. At the same time, some authors have formulated critiques of them. For example, in the forthcoming volume that Andreas De Block and I have edited on the experimental philosophy of disease, Maël Lemoine and Simon Okholm argue (in chapter 5) that to know the proper definition of disease, we should not investigate our intuitions as philosophers. Neither should we use surveys such as vignette studies to determine what laypeople think a disease is. Lemoine argues there is a whole range of definitions in the literature, and if we want a proper understanding of what is a disease and what is not, we must query that literature. Many of these discussions ignore one crucial aspect of how language works. With Stegenga, I agree that both normative and naturalist elements of disease are essential.

Also, in patients' experience, disease is more than the diagnosis but is a lived condition. The biological link is a necessary part of the disease experience. If someone feels deadly tired for months after having experienced a COVID-19 infection, the fact that this can be attributed to that infection matters for a whole range of actors. In the first place, it matters for the sufferer, as it substantiates the experience. It may matter for biomedical researchers who can now consider long COVID-19 a valid entry point for research into fatigue. It often matters for employers who are looking for proof of actual disease. We may think that is unfair. I agree that what matters most is the illness experience. However, that does not mean we should ignore how conceptualizations of symptoms and causation contribute to meaning.

Maybe we should not merely look at what a disease *is* but at how a phenomenon is created *as a disease* through different actors and practices. Leen De Vreese has argued for a *pragmatic approach* to disease (De Vreese, 2017). This entails describing how we build, use, apply and change our disease concept rather than trying to determine the proper definition of disease through conceptual analysis. 'Disease' is a practical concept that nonetheless plays a vital role in healthcare-related research and clinical decision-making processes (De Vreese, 2017). I think that even a simple question, 'Is phenomenon X a disease?' is not merely asking for an opinion on disease status. The person uttering this sentence is judging a phenomenon: we *should* call this a disease. Whether they think so may be based on different things, including a supposed biological cause, whether they consider this a bad thing to have, or whether it is a valid reason to take a day off from work. The answer may not only depend on the speaker's opinion. It also means investigating how we have used the concept of disease in bioethical thinking. Given the ethical implications of calling something a disease, analysing such networks of meaning, historically and contextually, is part and parcel of the task of the bioethicist.

Disability

When we single out 'disease' as a concept to be investigated using conceptual analysis or experimental philosophy, we often lose sight that it is associated with several other words, such as illness, disorder, and disability. Understanding the pragmatics of disability is especially relevant for bioethicists, as disability figures so prominently in many discussions on medical technologies and reproductive technologies. In mainstream bioethics, disability often carries the same negative connotation as *disease*: avoiding disability and disease seems to be the main aim of biomedical science, and bioethicists ensure that this happens ethically. Van Rensselaer Potter, for instance, believes it is better not to have a disabled child. For him, the main bioethical concern is overpopulation. His view is that if population growth is unavoidable, then we should at least make sure children are born without any disabilities. He argues for the termination of pregnancies where abnormalities are found: 'What if they were told that for the type of defect at hand, the next pregnancy would probably yield a normal child?' (Potter, 1988) This apparently stems from his experience that state institutions are 'hell' and, therefore, the quality of life of people in such places is minimal. Remarkably, creating a disability-friendly future does not seem to cross his mind.

When we look at disability as a concept, we must acknowledge its polysemic aspects. Disability, as a term, can be used as a synonym of disease: 'long COVID-19 is a debilitating disease', or 'long COVID-19 is a debilitating disability'. Nowadays, disability is used increasingly as the antonym of disease. Having spent many years of my academic career thinking about conceptualizations of autism, I have noticed how phenomena that may once have been conceptualized as diseases are now disabilities. Fifteen years ago, autism was sometimes still referred to as a 'devastating disease' in scientific literature. Today we consider it a disability, explicitly not a disease. Disability as a term has far more emancipating potential than 'disease'. Indeed, in recent years, disability scholars, philosophers, and activists have pointed out that the assumption, often made in the bioethics literature, that disabilities are necessarily bad to have, and to be avoided, is ableist, as it suggests that a disabled life is not worth living. The medical model of disability assumes that it should be prevented or treated. However, there is another way of thinking. For example, the social model states that the 'wrongs' of disability have less to do with the specific embodiment or cognitive reasoning and more with a lack of social support. Accommodation of disability rather than therapy is then the most appropriate answer. Philosopher Elizabeth Barnes has stated that having a disabled body is having a minority body (Barnes, 2016). Disability in itself is not good or bad. It is value-neutral. That is not to say that some people may not suffer from their specific disability, but disability is not automatically and straightforwardly harmful (Barnes, 2016). Crip theory also challenges traditional concepts of disability as straightforwardly related to lesser well-being and resists normalization and exclusion of specific others that do not fit within the paradigm of the normal (Kafer, 2013). Crip theory is not about a fixed disabled identity. It argues for a dynamic concept of disability and the inclusion of embodied experiences. Thus, it also challenges discourses of disability that present it as either too bleak or too rosy (the 'supercrip'). Instead, it asks us to imagine a world where disability is welcomed as a necessary part of diversity, not merely accommodated (Vanaken, 2022).

Engaging with philosophical accounts of disability, such as the philosophical account of Elizabeth Barnes and crip theory, which originated in the humanities, is of utmost importance for bioethicists. When confronted with ways of thinking that do not automatically link disability with being worse off and with empirical findings that suggest that disabled people do consider their lives pretty good, people often think this is counter-intuitive. Philosophers have even called it a paradox, the 'disability paradox'. However, disability scholars have pointed out that it is ableist even to consider this a paradox: it is proof of a lack of imagination on the part of non-disabled people that they cannot imagine disability and the good life together. As bioethicist Jackie Leach Scully argues in her brilliant book *Disability Bioethics*, bioethicists should actively engage with lived experiences of those who are disabled: 'the organic reality of the body and its processes is important to abstract thinking, including thinking about ethics' (Scully, 2008). In her thought-provoking book *Caring for my Daughter*, philosopher Eva Kittay, herself a mother of a daughter with an intellectual disability, describes 'the myth of independency', the idea that conceptions of a valuable life that hinge on factors such as independence and autonomy are misguided (Kittay, 2019). She stresses the centrality of care of interdependency. Not rationality, but joy, love, and attachment are at the centre of a valuable life. Thus, she challenges the conceptual scheme that underlies how bioethicists approach ethical dilemmas such as triage decisions. Looking at disability differently, and thinking with disability, will help avoid falling back to a default ableist stance during disasters like the COVID-19 pandemic. Joseph A. Stramondo points out, in his article *Tragic Choices: Disability, Triage, and Equity Amidst a Global Pandemic* (Stramondo, 2021), that who should be prioritized in triage discussions have often relied on the third-person quality of life judgments to deprioritize disabled or chronically ill people. Indeed, when push comes to shove, we often fall back to 'all things considered' or 'everything else being equal' judgements that switch the balance favouring non-disabled people when it comes to the survival lottery. Stramondo argues convincingly that the equation of health with well-being is often unjustified. In any case, it is not a general rule. Moreover, even by presenting such choices as 'tragic', we give the impression that there are no alternatives. Stramondo states, quoting disability scholar Shelley Tremain, that this means there should be structural efforts to ensure that we do not end up in the situation where we end up in such a 'tragic choice' in the first place (Stramondo, 2021). For bioethicists, such an approach implies that we must champion forward-looking policies that help ensure a future where all can thrive. At the same time, rather than quickly calling something that we cannot understand a 'paradox', we should do our utmost to try to understand.

Canguilhem and The World-Making of Disease Judgements

In the previous paragraphs, I explained some difficulties in pinning down disease and disability. I suggested a hybrid approach to disease, which acknowledges both a biological underpinning and an evaluative component, as a good step forward. At the same time, there is a performative aspect to disease: by calling a phenomenon a disease, we also insist that it is something bad. Considering the critique from many disability theorists, we realize that health and, specifically, non-disability should not be automatically linked with more well-being. Being able to flourish depends on factors within an individual and their relationship with others and the environment. This idea may be pretty straightforward when considering conditions that we consider 'mental' or 'psychological', or even 'neurodevelopmental'. Think about the person with ADHD who can use their specific characteristics to their advantage if provided with an environment that accommodates their atypical concentration span. In this chapter, I describe an approach to pathology that goes beyond the dualism of naturalism versus normativism and even hybridism and that acknowledges the normativism and creativity of life itself.

The ideas of French medical doctor and philosopher Georges Canguilhem provide a way of looking at disease that is neither dualist nor reductionist. Because it considers the entanglements of organisms and milieu, such a vision demands a renewed interest in individual experiences rather than a mere focus on looking for 'biological causes'.

At the same time, focusing on experiences and values does not imply that diseases should be seen as 'all in the head'. Clinicians and alternative medicine practitioners often make this associative mistake. Clinicians demand a cause or symptom to make a diagnosis, while the latter decries traditional medicine and claims that 'minds' can heal 'bodies'. Clinicians may send a patient home with the message that nothing is wrong because the blood test results were OK. I am thinking of a discussion on social media I witnessed about vaccination. A specific person argued that diseases are not harmful and it is possible to overcome them by healing the mind of trauma. Contrary to the claims of holistic medicine, many alternative practitioners start from the same dualistic mind-body reductionism as classical medicine. This time it is the mind that can control the body. However, thinking with Georges Canguilhem, we can take a non-reductionist view on biology as a starting point. In this view, we do not assume that specific symptoms are more easily cured by medicine or alternative treatments. Neither does it mean that fatigue, for example, without a particular cause, is necessarily 'in the head'. In light of the uncertainty and perhaps even indeterminacy of the concept of a 'real' disease, the most prudent thing to do may be to take people's words at face value. At the same time, by classifying something as a disease, we also change experiences, both those of patients and those of clinicians. Classifying is world-making and life-altering. I will come back to that later on.

So, who was this Georges Canguilhem, to whom I seem to return in much of my writing? Canguilhem was a medical doctor and philosopher arguing that illness and pathology are to be found in an individual's relation with the environment or milieu rather than in characteristics of the structures or behaviours that we consider sick:

> There is no objective pathology. Structures or behaviours can be objectively described but they cannot be called 'pathological' on the strength of some purely objective criterion. Objectively, only varieties or differences can be defined with positive or negative vital values. (Canguilhem, 1989)

Canguilhem considers the pathological as a different kind of 'normal', a condition that can stand independently and where other norms prevail. He gives the example of diabetes: this involves not merely statistically higher glucose levels in the body, but the cooperation of different factors.

The circulatory, nervous, and endocrine systems all react differently to changes in movement or food. As a result, the normal state can no longer function as the checkpoint to see whether something is normal or pathological. Therefore, attempts such as those of Christopher Boorse, aiming at pinpointing a generalizable way of looking at pathology, are doomed to fail.

> If the normal does not have the rigidity of a fact of collective constraint, but rather the flexibility of a norm which is transformed in its relation to individual conditions, it is clear that the boundary between the normal and the pathological becomes imprecise. (Canguilhem, 1989)

Canguilhem introduces the concept of *biological normativity*, a normativity in relation to the environmental and historical context (Giroux, 2019). Organisms adapt to their environment or try to adapt to their environment to survive in it. *Health* is the margin of tolerance to change:

> Being healthy means being not only normal in a given situation, but also normative in this and other eventual [sic] situations. What characterizes health is the possibility of transcending the norm, which defines the momentary normal, the possibility of tolerating infractions of the habitual normal and instituting new norms in new situations. [...] Health is a margin of tolerance for the inconstancies of the environment. (Canguilhem, 1989)

Canguilhem talks about propulsive norms—when the organism can define new norms and adapt to new circumstances—and about repulsive norms when this is no longer possible. The organism must struggle to maintain itself. *Pathology* is a negative biological *experience*: Thinking of our bodies as an organism, we perceive ourselves to be ill if that organism is less resistant to changes (repulsive). There may be an objective explanation of where the mismatch lies, but disease and health are located at the level of experience. They are necessarily relational. As such, 'disease' cannot be objectified by science. Medicine, to Canguilhem, is more of an art than a science. Hence, what medical doctors must do is listen to experiences of suffering.

Although the traditions in which Canguilhem's ideas arose and the ideas I have sketched in chapters 1 and 2 are different, I believe Canguilhem's approach complements these ideas. It is a biological approach, albeit not a reductionist one. It is easy to see how normativism can also be considered constructivism and how, in this view, only human beings can be genuinely ill, as human values are at stake. However, although Canguilhem was a medical doctor taking care of human beings, the view of health and pathology as the interaction and even entanglement of well-being and the environment that Canguilhem sketches apply to many organisms. If we think that experience is available in many forms of life, so is, unfortunately, also the experience of illness. Hence, we open up a view on posthumanist pathology, which entails an ethical appeal to care for ill humans, other-than-human beings, and maybe even ill environments. Also, it is a call to take experiences seriously. There is no need to judge someone's testimonial based on whatever biomarkers we find. Although biomarkers and lesions can help make sense of an experience, they are not needed as validation, assuming the subject is telling the truth. It also means that what matters for research is what is experienced in a specific context in space and time. A research practice inspired by Canguilhem thus entails idiosyncratic descriptions of cases and experiences as much as generalizable data. Moreover, the 'solution' to illness lies as much in the environment as in the organism. Anna Bosman gives an example of approaches to ADHD that emphasize environmental interventions—allowing children to get up and move in classrooms—alongside prescription medicine (Bosman, 2017). Environmental relativity also means the physical environment: think about epigenetics and pollution. Indeed, it would be nonsensical, in my view, to consider biomedical ethics and environmental ethics separately.

Norms and diseases are also linked differently. Normativism and constructionism are often thought of as the opposite of naturalism: diseases are what we suffer from and value negatively, rather than something that has an essence in biology. Nevertheless, calling something a disease is also a speech act. By saying something like 'poverty is a disease' or even 'fatigue is a disease', we not only suggest that it satisfies the conditions of the concept of disease, be they evaluative or naturalist, but we also suggest that we think it should be classified, and therefore treated, as something we do not want and should try to remedy. Indeed, the seemingly unsurmountable difficulty of grasping what a disease is through conceptual analysis suggests that it may be impossible to find the final answer to what is truly a disease. Some scholars, including Elizabeth Grosz following Gilles Deleuze and Félix Guattari, have generally questioned the idea of a concept as something that can be pinned down. In *Becoming Undone*, Grosz writes that

> Concepts emerge, have value and function only through the impact of problems generated from the outside. [...] Concepts are not solutions to problems, for most problems — the problem of gravity, of living with others, of mortality, of the weather — have no solutions, only ways of living with problems. (Grosz, 2011, p. 78)

Disease judgement may be a problem that cannot be solved by getting the concept right. Rather than describing a phenomenon, a disease judgment reinforces the idea that the phenomenon should be considered a disease or something undesirable. Hence, calling something 'disease' is also *making it a disease*. This disease-making is not good or bad per se, but it is morally relevant. Considering something as a disease can benefit those suffering from the phenomenon, giving credibility to their suffering. It relieves sufferers from blame or from being seen as weak. It justifies sick leave and reimbursement. If we consider long COVID-19 as an actual disease, this opens up possibilities for research into treatments.

Nevertheless, it is not always straightforwardly good to be considered 'a patient'. Think about a phenomenon such as ADHD. On the one hand, denying that ADHD is a 'real disorder' may lead to people missing out on medication that can vastly improve their well-being. On the other hand, looking at ADHD as merely a disease to be 'solved' misses out on the possibility of seeing it as a unique, worthwhile, albeit sometimes troubling, way of being. By associating ADHD with disorder or disease, we create a world where this is the primary lens through which it is seen. This lens creates both opportunities for research funding for causes and genes and closes down different ways of looking. Ultimately, I think we are misguided if we solely focus on whether we have classified something rightly or wrongly as a disease. It is equally important to consider the diseases and consider what we create by classification. Classification is not morally wrong per se, but it is morally relevant to consider its consequences.

The Strange Case of Human Enhancement

Whether we consider something pathological or not has normative weight in the debate on medicalization, we do not want to classify something as a disease when it is not. The distinction between therapy and enhancement seems to carry normative weight as well. For example, for many, it is intuitively allowed to use genetic technologies to avoid diseases in future offspring but not to enhance the traits of people. In what follows, I take a closer look at the presuppositions of the enhancement debate.

In 2011 I started a postdoctoral project at the University of Maastricht in reproductive ethics, specifically the issue of comprehensive chromosome screening of *in vitro* embryos. The questions we sought to answer in that project were related to embryo selection based on genetic information gathered from these embryos during an IVF procedure. For example, on which basis should we choose one embryo over another? What does it mean for an embryo to have 'better genes' than another one? Genetic technologies that were relatively new, such as whole-genome sequencing and analysis, and microarray screening, would allow embryologists to learn much more about the genetic makeup than previously thought. That couples who were carriers of a specific genetic mutation such as cystic fibrosis would want to use preimplantation diagnosis and IVF to pick an embryo without that specific mutation seemed straightforward, provided you did not see any problem with the fact that embryos carrying a mutation would be discarded. However, the possibility of finding other genetic information raised questions as to how to act on that information. Intuitively, it seemed that there was a scale of acceptability: making selections based on genetic mutations for known genetic diseases seemed far less morally problematic than selections based on late-onset diseases or even traits considered non-medical, such as eye colours. In 2011, we thought the focus should be on embryo selection, as this technique was proven to work. The idea that embryologists could manipulate the genes of an embryo we considered science fiction: the science simply was not available yet. However, in 2012, CRISPR/Cas9 technology was discovered. This technique allowed for the relatively cheap and straightforward manipulation of genes in different organisms. People started to speculate about using the technology *in vitro* embryos. In this way, it could be an alternative to embryo selection, for example, if not enough embryos were available *in vitro* to choose from. In principle, the editing of genes in embryos was proved possible and has been demonstrated by a study in 2015 on non-viable embryos. Researchers edited the gene responsible for beta-thalassemia. In April 2016, researchers managed to edit a gene linked to HIV resistance again in non-viable embryos. CRISPR/Cas9 was deemed revolutionary for work in plants and somatic cells from human and other-than-human embryos. Nevertheless, most researchers considered it either too early or undesirable altogether to use the techniques in embryos that would be used for reproductive purposes.

Fast forward to 2018, when the world was shocked by the announcement that the first genetically altered babies were born. The researcher responsible for the experiment, He Jiankui, stated that two babies, Lulu and Nana, had their genomes modified when they were *in vitro* embryos to introduce a mutation that makes them resistant to HIV infection. Being HIV positive is associated with much stigma and discrimination in the region of China where He performed the procedure. Nana and Lulu's father was HIV positive, and it is claimed that he wanted to prevent his children from facing the same stigma. He Jiankui was denounced for having violated many rules of research ethics. At the writing of this book, he is serving a sentence in prison. It is easy to see him as a kind of Frankenstein scientist. However, in the video 'About Lulu and Nana', Jiankui explains his motives.[1] He is adamant that he did not develop the procedure to raise a future child's IQ or eye colour. He stresses that the technology should only be used for 'healing'. It is a procedure that would only apply to a tiny subset of parents, for whom this is the only option to give their child an equal chance at a healthy life. He gives the example of cystic fibrosis, a heritable genetic disease, as a good application for the genetic modification of embryos.

Nevertheless, it is remarkable that the changes he introduced in the embryos made them resistant to HIV. To many, introducing such resistance is not the same as 'healing' an embryo so that it is not born with a specific congenital disease. HIV is preventable through other means, and the resulting children may never run the risk of being infected by HIV. HIV

---

1   https://www.youtube.com/watch?v=th0vnOmFltc

prevention seems to situate itself on the fine line between therapy and enhancement. Would we judge it closer to changing one's eye colour or 'removing' a cystic fibrosis gene? Interestingly, we could argue that it is precisely in the case of enhancement that genetic modification comes in handy. In many instances in which both prospective parents are carriers of a genetic mutation for a recessive disease like cystic fibrosis, embryo selection procedures will be sufficient. However, suppose we want to introduce an 'improved' gene. We cannot work with the available genetic material, and genetic modification using techniques such as CRISPR/Cas might be the only option. Nevertheless, the idea of enhancement will make many uncomfortable. In what follows, I shall briefly sketch the debate on enhancement and introduce transhumanist thinking. After that, I shall zoom in on two philosophical questions that arise: what is 'a better life' and the question of what kind of view of human nature is at the core of the enhancement/transhumanist debate. To do so, I will juxtapose 'transhumanism' and the idea of 'the posthuman' with philosophical or critical posthumanism.

It seems straightforward that medical technologies with a primarily therapeutic purpose are far less morally problematic than those that somehow improve a specific characteristic. In reproductive ethics, enhancement is sometimes used as an example to draw the line with regard to which genetic manipulations we are allowed to perform on an embryo. For instance, we have relatively liberal legislation for embryo experimentation in Belgium. It is allowed to use *in vitro* embryos in biomedical experiments and even create embryos for that purpose. At the same time, there are many restrictions. One of the restrictions is that this cannot be done for eugenic purposes. Article 5, number 4 in the law regarding research on embryos *in vitro* (law of 11 May 2003, law concerning the research on embryos *in vitro*) states that:

> Het is verboden: Onderzoek of behandelingen met een eugenetisch oogmerk uit te voeren, dit wil zeggen gericht op de selectie of de verbetering van niet-pathologische genetische kenmerken van de menselijke soort.

Translated, this reads

> that it is forbidden to perform research or treatment with a eugenic aim, which means: with the aim of the selection or improvement of non-pathological genetic characteristic of the human species.

This quote shows that enhancement through medical procedures and technologies is closely associated with eugenics. Enhancement commonly refers to the bettering, in this case, of human beings. We can think about removing diseases from the gene pool and increasing longevity, making people more skilled musically, physically, or cognitively. Some people have also argued that we should make people more moral, social, and productive if these traits would have a primary genetic basis. Eugenics, broadly conceived, refers to the genetic enhancement of an individual, the human race or a specific people. Although eugenic thinking neither started nor stopped with the Nazis, it is still often associated with their endeavours to create a 'better people' and, therefore, morally suspect. At the same time, authors such as Nicholas Agar have argued that we should disassociate eugenics from the Nazis (Agar, 2008). After all, the Nazis tried to create a 'better' race, which is far worse than specific parents wanting to give a child a head start in life. Some commentators have argued that we could even see the latter as an example of good parenting. In such 'new' or 'liberal' eugenics, the initiative does not come from the state but is chosen by individuals, for example, parents who choose characteristics for their children (Agar, 2008). This is far less morally suspect for some ethicists and could even be considered morally good. For example, Oxford philosopher Julian Savulescu has argued for a 'principle of procreative beneficence': if parents, in the context of embryo selection, can choose an embryo that is expected to live a better life than the other embryos, parents have a good reason, perhaps even a moral duty to do so. Savulescu argues that this applies to avoiding diseases and includes promoting genes that supposedly make one's life better. For example, if you happen to have an embryo with very 'smart' genes, you should select that one (Savulescu and Kahane, 2009). He gives the example of an embryo with a potential IQ of 140. Procreative beneficence is *a consequentialist principle*. It has to do with the consequences for the future child. Others have used arguments based on parents' right to reproductive autonomy to choose their future children's genes. Such arguments are rights-based or deontological arguments. Those favouring genetic techniques to enhance future children's characteristics often argue that biomedical technologies are not that different from what we have always done in raising children. After all, we often choose partners to reproduce with based on specific characteristics. In many places, the fact that we now have better food and better hygiene has contributed to our longevity.

Opponents of genetic enhancement through biomedical technologies argue a fundamental difference. Choosing or changing genes is often compared to 'playing God'. For some, this is to be taken quite literally: it is their religious conviction that creation is good as it is, and we may not tamper with it. Others refer to the inherent dignity that human beings have, and changing or choosing genes is then considered a form of instrumentalisation. Nevertheless, secular arguments can also be of the 'playing God' type. In my bioethics course, sometimes students argue that manipulating genes disturbs the natural working of evolution and is, therefore, harmful.

Other opponents point out that such technologies would lead to structural inequality and medicine for the rich. There may be a rift between those with good genes and those who do not have good genes. Such interventions would effectively create an underclass of non-enhanced people at the mercy of the posthuman class. Also, these technologies may be too dangerous to develop. After all, if we want to test whether these technologies are safe for humans, we have no other choice than to create said humans. In light of current superwicked problems related to pandemics, global poverty, and climate change, we may wonder whether any other issues require our attention and money first. Should we invest in research into making people more intelligent or with more memory, given that our world has been turned upside down by something seemingly trivial as an infectious disease? Even before the pandemic, at the inception of the transhumanist movement, the relative biomedical comfort from which these ideas could have been written was only available to countries in the Global North. I will not delve into these questions now, but I want to tackle two philosophical questions in the rest of the chapter. The first question relates to whether we can pinpoint 'improvement'. The second question is, what view on human beings do enhancement advocates have and is this view correct.

However, before we go there, let us first consider some of the most outspoken advocates for enhancement: the transhumanists and their desire to reach a 'posthuman' stage. Genetic manipulation and technological advancements are part and parcel of thinking about transhumanism. Transhumanism is the idea that humanity should take its destiny into its own hands. Transhumanists argue that we should invest in biomedical technologies to increase longevity, make us smarter, and enhance our overall memory capacity and quality of life. It is characterised by a strong belief that technology will accomplish this. Oxford philosopher and transhumanist Nick Bostrom describes it as follows:

> Transhumanism is a loosely defined movement that has developed gradually over the past two decades, and can be viewed as an outgrowth of secular humanism and the Enlightenment. It holds that current human nature is improvable through the use of applied science and other rational methods, which may make it possible to increase human health span, extend our intellectual and physical capacities, and give us increased control over our own mental states and moods. (Bostrom, 2005)

According to Bostrom, opponents to the idea that humanity should enhance itself suffer from a *status quo bias*: 'an inappropriate, (irrational) preference for an option because it preserves the status quo' (Bostrom and Ord, 2006). From a utilitarian perspective, preserving the status quo is nonsense, as biomedical technologies will enable us to make life better for humankind. Of course, Bostrom states, we would want to make people more intelligent, just as we would vehemently oppose a toxin that would decrease our IQ.

According to transhumanists, enhancement should be accomplished via futuristic technologies such as genetic manipulation or the integration of computers into brains. In the meantime, bodies can be preserved using cryogenic technologies to wait, after death, for a future where there will be no more death. Indeed, technological advancements will eventually generate such enhanced human beings that will be so different to us that they can be considered a different species. This will be our 'posthuman future'. As Max More, one well-known transhumanist who investigates cryopreservation, states:

> Physically, we will have become posthuman only when we have made such fundamental and sweeping modifications to our inherited genetics, physiology, neurophysiology and neurochemistry that we can no longer be usefully classified with Homo Sapiens. (More, 1994)

The terms 'enhancement' and 'eugenics' imply that we can easily find out what is better. Transhumanists assumed that having higher intelligence, better social skills, better memory, and an extended lifespan are traits to be desired. Suppose you are an Oxford professor enjoying your cognitive skills. In that case, it may indeed be understandable that you assume that cognitive skills are directly related to a good life and well-being. In the case of parents choosing in place of their children, it becomes more tricky. They may think that cognitively strong children are happier in the end or believe it adds to their prestige if the child performs well at school. And indeed, it is so that in many societies nowadays, intellectual skill is in higher regard than technical skill, which may contribute to the well-being of people with good cognitive skills. However, by sustaining the discourse surrounding cognitive skills in discussions about embryo selection, we are also maintaining the idea that cognitive skills are what matters. Another example one sometimes hears in discussions is that of perfect pitch. Some people may want a child with a gene that enhances the child's musical abilities. Whether having a perfect pitch increases the chance that the child has a good life is highly dependent on the hopes and dreams of the child in question. Examples from theory and literature challenge the assumption that defining a good or a better life is easy. In the comic book *Watchmen* (Wieseler, 2020), Dr Manhattan is a scientist who, through a freak accident, has become a superhuman with excessive cognitive skills(*Watchmen*, 2008). However, this makes him lonely: his girlfriend leaves him to be with a more mundane partner. In Simone De Beauvoir's book *Tous les hommes sont mortels*, a man has gained immortality and has lived for ages (de Beauvoir, 2015). De Beauvoir describes the utter boredom the protagonist experiences. In *The Evolution of the Sensitive Soul*, Simona Ginsburg and Eva Jablonka explain how 'forgetting' is an equally important aspect of being conscious. The possibility to forget has evolved alongside the ability to remember precisely because memories can also be harmful and traumatizing.

It may be more worthwhile to imagine a society where diversity is celebrated and where flourishing is not dependent on nor immediately associated with specific cognitive or other skills that happened to be deemed valuable at a certain point in history. David Boden and Sarah Chan have argued that enhancement imaginaries in bioethics reinforce already available concepts of normalcy, of 'species typical functioning' (Boden and Chan, 2022). Even if, at first sight, enhancement enthusiasts reject the normative boundaries between therapy and enhancement, they accept implicitly the underlying assumption that 'normal' is a point or a range on a linear, directional spectrum movement along which is necessarily worse in one direction, better in the other. (Boden and Chan, 2022, p. 30)

As well as it being difficult to identify the characteristics that would make our lives better, it also seems complicated to draw a line between disease and enhancement. We have seen that this distinction carries normative weight. It seems essential to make this distinction because, intuitively, many would think that employing biomedical technology to cure people (make people better) is less problematic than using it to make better people. However, defining disease is complex using only universal and objective grounds. Does someone with mild symptoms of COVID-19 have 'the disease' COVID-19? Is ADHD a disease? As Michael Wee describes, the advent of preventive medicine is a case in point: how to classify, for example, vaccination, a practice that we think is firmly part of medicine? Is this enhancement or treatment? (Wee, 2022) As we have seen before, philosophers have tried to lay down objective characteristics of what makes a disease, for example, based on statistics or evolution. For me, these are all unconvincing. We may want to define disease as what causes us suffering, as some normativists have tried. This would mean that what we consider 'disease' or a neutral trait is highly context-dependent, and so is the distinction between therapy and enhancement. I have also described the views of Georges Canguilhem. He states that pathology is the suffering we (or an organism) experience if we can no longer adapt our environment to our needs. Pathology is related to our specific milieu and is not (solely) an intrinsic feature of an individual. If we go back to the case of Lulu and Nana, who were genetically modified to be HIV-resistant, some would probably consider this an example of enhancement. However, this was different for those living in that Chinese region, as HIV was associated with much stigma. Alternatively, think about our current situation: Suppose there would be a gene technology to introduce COVID-19 resistance into embryos. We would probably not advocate that future children undergo this as an embryo right now. However, we can imagine a bleak future where another pandemic has wreaked such havoc on the world that many would deem this acceptable.

As I pointed out earlier, disability scholars and crip theorists and activists have challenged the idea that disability is automatically linked to a worse life. Bioethicists often share the view that a diverse society in which disabled people feel at home is valuable and worthy of consideration. Here, we bump into one of the inconsistencies of much reasoning surrounding transhumanism. Many transhumanists are also libertarians: it is about the right to choose a better intelligence or an eternal life for oneself and one's children. But as David Boden and Sarah Chan have demonstrated, there is an inconsistency here:

> While arguments supporting the permissibility of enhancement may have originated in liberal humanist ideals of freedom to pursue a 'good life' by whatever means available, including technological, the arguments for an obligation to enhance tend towards the coercive in their normative visions of what 'a good life' might entail and, especially, what the biomedical preconditions of such a life might be. (Boden and Chan, 2022, p. 30)

Indeed, there is the assumption that it is possible to set what is best for everyone in stone. By assuming that there is a list of characteristics that are straightforwardly linked to a good life, I think we mistake confounding the good life of an individual with what might be considered 'good' for society. We could assume that people with exceptional abilities will produce many good outcomes for the community, such as medical improvements or solutions to climate challenges. Moreover, whether being selected for intelligence for the good of humanity is better for the enhanced persons themselves remains to be seen. It is also uncertain whether they would feel inclined to use their capabilities for the people's good. There is no guarantee that a clever person will be altruistic. Unless there is a crowd of people sharing the same enhancements, being an enhanced human being seems a lonely place. Suppose we use arguments relating to the good such individuals bring to society. In that case, we must be prepared to tackle tricky questions regarding the acceptability of creating human beings with specific characteristics for the sake of humanity. This is no longer 'liberal eugenics'. Instead, I would argue that defining the good life cannot be done 'in the abstract', based on characteristics such as intelligence and memory and so on. In order to determine the good life, life must be lived. 'Living well' means living in a specific context in which you and your characteristics are cherished and welcomed, whatever they are. It has to do with having valuable relations, taking care and being taken care of, and joy. Using enhancement technologies to enhance specific characteristics in yourself that you value may perfectly align with that vision. Deciding a priori what could be a good life for children that have not been born yet may be misguided. Nevertheless, it is natural to want the best for one's children, even if we can never be sure what that means.

Besides the very private sphere of human reproduction, human enhancement debates have also entered discussions about our current environmental crises. Humanity is facing unprecedented challenges. We are hitting our planet's boundaries hard regarding environmental damage, climate change, and biodiversity loss (Rockström *et al.*, 2009). We can distinguish two opposite visions on how we can tackle these issues. On the one hand, ecomodernists often share the same mindset as transhumanists. They believe that science and technology can save us. On the other hand, bioconservationists argue that we should return to a more natural, less consumerist version of living. We have become estranged from ourselves, and this estrangement, partly to blame on technology, has led us to our current predicament. Also, genetic technologies have entered the discussion. With genetic technologies, some have argued, we can change ourselves because of the environmental changes we face. We can, for example, use CRISPR/Cas9 on our epigenome to 'scissor away' the impact of pollution. Alternatively, we can genetically modify people, for example, to mitigate their effect on the environment by making them smaller. Alternatively, we can make them more resilient against the upcoming environmental challenges. They could be more able to withstand the heat or digest food that can withstand the heat. Others, such as Francis Fukuyama, see 'human nature' as something that cannot be touched. He states that

> human nature, as 'the sum of the behaviour and characteristics typical of the human species, arising from genetic rather than environmental factors', is a guiding principle and that any genetic technologies would unacceptably change human nature. (Fukuyama, 2002)

Nevertheless, both those who think that human nature should be changed for the better or that it should be left untouched hold a shared belief that there is such a thing as an intrinsic human nature: an atomistic core that can either be changed or left alone. The same idea is present in transhumanism, which endeavours to transcend humanism. Transhumanists often think we can manipulate ourselves to become something else if we use our rationality and science. Humans are simultaneously an object being manipulated as subjects that do the manipulation. This ties in with 20th-century views on genetics. Think about the metaphors of our genes as a book of life, the blueprint from which we are built. This view on genetics goes hand in hand with the development of cybernetics in the mid-20th century. People increasingly began to see the brain as a computer and the 'mind' as software that runs on that hardware. I think, however, based on recent findings in biology (and maybe also on ancient knowledge), that this vision is not entirely correct. We have already seen the ideas of Georges Canguilhem, who considers the interactions of organisms and their experiences as central. Several findings and theoretical assumptions in systems biology prove this is correct. For example, the gut has been called 'the second brain': our microbiome influences our moods and personalities. In her book *Gut Feminism*, Elizabeth Wilson argues that the gut may even be considered an 'organ of the mind' (Wilson, 2015). Moreover, this microbiome is closely linked to our environment and lifestyle (Ahmed and Hens, 2021). Recent findings in evolutionary biology challenge the idea that genes are passed on only vertically through the generations. Genes can jump within and between organisms; such jumping genes may cause new species to arise.

The transhumanists defined the posthuman as a being so far enhanced that it is no longer considered part of the species homo sapiens. As Danielle Sands explains, it is an 'intensification of humanism, combining the enlightenment valorisation of scientific rationality with a commitment to technologies which promise liberation from perceived disorders and deficiencies, and even, perhaps, death' (Sands, 2022, p. 2). However, in the last decades, posthumanism also has a different meaning, a meaning that is perhaps even antonymic to the one that the transhumanists gave it (Sands, 2022). Critical posthumanism 'looks to identify, resist and disrupt mastery at all levels.... It is particularly alert to the stabilisation, naturalisation or appropriation of the figure of the "human," turning its focus on the contexts, networks and entanglements from which it emerges' (Sands, 2022, p. 3).

Think about Donna Haraway's cyborg metaphor. For Haraway, the cyborg does not transcend human nature, but human beings are always cyborgs: hybrid creatures. Her seminal text, *A Cyborg Manifesto*, urges the reader to think beyond dualisms between man-woman, nature-culture and nature-technology (Haraway, 1991). In recent posthumanist thinking, relationality is pivotal: we are not solely individuals. We relate to other humans, other-than-humans, and the physical environment. In this way, it offers a different view than the 'back to nature' of deep ecologists, and at the same time, it is not a technological optimism. For example, in their overview article, Keeling and Lehman write:

> Whereas a humanist perspective frequently assumes the human is an autonomous, conscious, and intentional actor with exceptional capabilities, a posthumanist perspective assumes the human's ability to act is distributed across a dynamic set of relationships that the human participates in but does not completely intend or control. The 'post' indicates a rethinking of the individualism and superiority of the human in our worldly relations, a position that is both intrinsic to many ancient and contemporary understandings of rhetoric and increasingly critiqued in contemporary communication studies. Posthumanist philosophy conceptualises the human as: (a) moved to action through a variety of environmental interactions, affects, habits and sometimes reasons; (b) physically, chemically, and biologically formed by and dependent on their environment; and (c) possessing no attribute that is uniquely human, but is instead made up of a larger evolving ecosystem. (Keeling and Lehman, 2018)

I believe a posthumanist conception of human nature fits well with system biology approaches. Such approaches also fit in with dynamic and normative biological concepts of pathology, which consider disease as lesions, infections or genetic mutations and entangled with the milieu in which an organism lives. This also means we make something a disease by calling something a disease. Our task is to make sure we think very hard about the world we want to create.

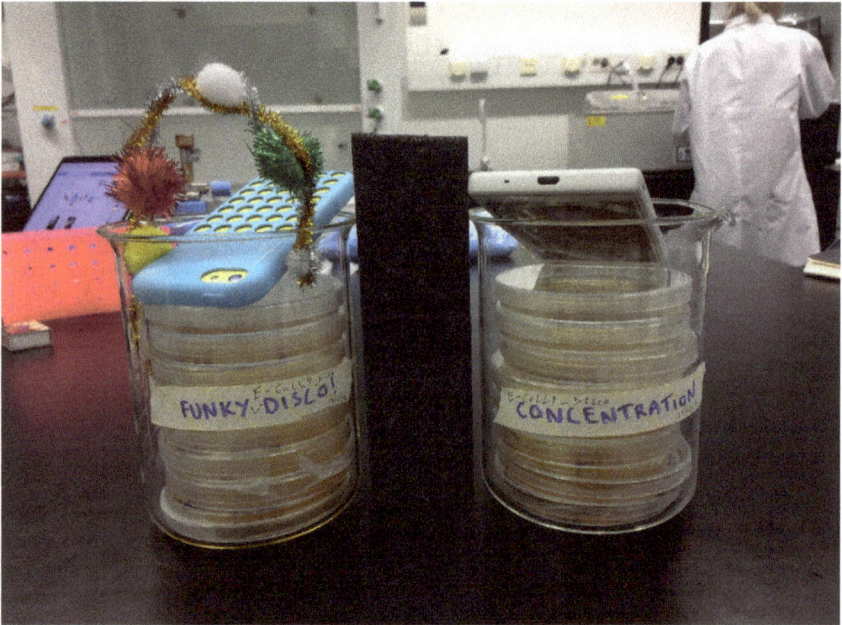

E. coli Funky Disco Concentration.
How to increase literacy on gene editing technologies like CRISPR-Cas9?
Object inspired by bacterial quorum sensing.
Photo by Bartaku, 2018[2]

---

2   Intuitive creation made during merryCRISPR 1 — the first of two workshops
     produced by the Finnish Bioart Society and Aalto ARTS, facilitated by
     Marta de Menezes. Biofilia, Lab for Biological Arts, Aalto University, 2018,
     https://bioartsociety.fi/posts/merry-crispr-workshop

12. Standpoints

In Part Two, I described a view on life that is fundamentally relational, situated in time. In the previous paragraphs, I argued for a perspective on disease relative to the environment. However, this does not mean that this is a one-way influence. Relationality is bidirectional. According to Canguilhem, health is as much about how the world shapes organisms as about the extent to which they can shape the world. However, such a relational view of knowledge and the world is also relevant to how we think about science and ethics. It means that there is no 'God Trick', in the words of Donna Haraway (Haraway, 1988). We cannot assume the position of an omniscient god when we do science, as all knowledge is situated. This does not mean that there is no such thing as objective science. It is easy to fall back to either relativism and think there can be no objective knowledge or positivism and even scientism: a denial that science is situated and that different standpoints yield different aspects of knowledge. Regarding ethical knowledge, we can find adherents to both extreme positions. Moral norms can be seen as either absolute or relative. They are considered universal and applicable everywhere or seen as relative to specific cultures and times. Bioethics has long acknowledged the importance of not only starting from general moral theories or principles but incorporating particular norms and values and situated knowledge in ethical decision-making. I contend it is an essential task of the bioethicist to ensure that situatedness is taken into account on all levels, in the science we are dealing with and in the ethical reflection about the science. Such an approach implies that ethicists and philosophers, together with other humanities and social sciences scholars, can take an essential role in life-sciences research to enable such an approach. At the same time, we also need a framework to argue for incorporating different standpoints in research. More and more, funding agencies are requesting that research proposals, especially when of a

 https://doi.org/10.11647/OBP.0320.12

clinical research kind, also describe how stakeholders will be engaged. In clinical research, especially, this has taken the form of advisory boards that consist of patient representatives and other stakeholders, such as parents and friends of patients. However, sometimes researchers consider the engagement of stakeholders as a tick-box exercise at best or as something that seriously hampers their research efforts at worst. Indeed, for more fundamental research into disease mechanisms, there is the fear that the requirement of patient engagement will ultimately divest from necessary basic research. I believe it is possible to argue for incorporating different standpoints in fundamental research in the life sciences. Such incorporation implies the acknowledgement that it is about the practical implications of research for patients and about having access to new ways of seeing realities, which are fundamentally situated. In what follows, I will draw from the rich corpus of theory that feminist epistemologists and ethicists have approached, formed, and incorporated in their many contributions to the *International Journal of Feminist Approaches to Bioethics* (*IJFAB: International Journal of Feminist Approaches to Bioethics*, no date). However, this corpus rarely found its way into mainstream bioethics, which often takes the ideal of neutral, 'view from nowhere' science for granted.

Epistemic Standpoints and Epistemic (In)Justices

It seems straightforward that patients are involved in developing applications based on clinical knowledge. After all, they are the ones who will be using them. To what extent people consider engaging stakeholders and querying different standpoints beneficial to the underlying science is unclear. Science is often thought to be neutral: only the scientific method will ensure that we find objective knowledge. Bothering the public will only lead to delays and worse science. However, since the nineties, feminist epistemologists have argued that to arrive at genuine or strong objectivity in science, it is necessary to include the standpoints of those belonging to marginalized groups. One of the champions of this *feminist standpoint epistemology* is Sandra Harding. She argues that the ideal of neutrality in science is not a solution that helps avoid political values getting entangled with scientific knowledge. Instead, neutrality, or objectivism, is the problem:

> Objectivism defends and legitimizes the institutions and practices through which the distortions and their often-exploitative consequences are generated. It certifies as value-neutral, normal, natural, and therefore not political at all the policies and practices through which powerful groups can gain the information and explanation that they need to advance their priorities. (Harding, 1995, p. 337)

Such 'weak objectivity' does not acknowledge science's partiality. Indeed, by assuming that the predominant scientific practice is the neutral and objective one, we forget that this science is done chiefly from the standpoint of the white male scientist or philosopher. It is androcentric. Harding writes: 'The Archimedean observer of good science is the impartial administrator of liberal political theory and the disinterested moral philosopher — the "good man" — of liberal ethics' (Harding, 1991, p. 58).

Of course, that does not mean this standpoint is wrong per se. It is just not the whole story. Think about the emphasis on competition in contemporary evolutionary theory and on the idea of genes that do everything to propagate subsequent generations. We have seen in Part Two that different approaches to life are possible—approaches that stress cooperation, chance and, as we shall see in Part Four, *Care*. Nevertheless, to perceive such complementary approaches to evolution, science must incorporate the standpoints of those not part of the dominant discourse. Harding's strong claim is that including the standpoints of marginalized groups, which are not typically associated with scientific practice, makes science better and more complete. It is not just nice to have:

> The history of science shows that research directed by maximally liberatory social interests and values tends to be better equipped to identify partial claims and distorting assumptions, even though the credibility of the scientists who do it may not be enhanced during the short run. After all, antiliberatory interests and values are invested in the natural inferiority of just the groups of humans who, if given realm equal access (not just the formally equal access that is liberalism's goal) to public voice, would most strongly contest claims about their purported natural inferiority. Antiliberatory interests and values silence and destroy the most likely sources of evidence against their own claims. That is what makes them rational for elites. (Harding, 1991, pp. 148–149)

Hence, Harding strongly argues that good science is always political because it is inclusive. It acknowledges that science is done from a specific cultural perspective, which can be wrong and biased. Including as many standpoints as possible helps objectivity and helps to unmask shared assumptions underlying knowledge.

The task of bioethics is to ensure that both fundamental and practical science is the best we can get. This means that advocating for the inclusion of different standpoints and visions is part and parcel of our job descriptions. It also means acknowledging that the distinction between 'pure' and applied sciences or technology is not as straightforward as commonly assumed. Fundamental science is already related to the application of science. It is not necessary to pinpoint a specific application when discovering certain fundamental truths to acknowledge that the discovery will, most of the time, have implications, although we may not be able to predict them. Moreover, as Sandra Harding has argued, standpoints and values play a role at the point of discovery. They influence what we conceive of as valid objects of investigation and what we conceive of as scientific. Consider the example of inductive risk, the chance that one will be wrong in accepting (or rejecting) a scientific hypothesis. Heather Douglas has argued convincingly that choosing what seems to be very technical statistical data, such as thresholds for significance, is value-laden (Douglas, 2000). Douglas gives the example of tests for toxicity levels in animals. The decision of what is statistically significant in delimiting toxic from non-toxic levels is not merely a scientific one: Non-epistemic values play a role in determining what is significant and what is not. Indeed, false positives will lead to policies that are excessively protective about which levels are acceptable. Ultimately such policies are more protective of public health risks. However, if the significance is set to tolerate more false negatives, the level that is considered safe is higher than it should be. Such a policy is less protective of public health. Still, it may be better for cost-effectiveness for the industry, which may value the fact that higher acceptable levels will enable more extensive use of the specific product. It is thus a mistake to assume that non-epistemic values do not play a role in science (Douglas, 2000).

Standpoint epistemology is not only relevant to exact sciences or applied sciences. It can also function as a framework for strong ethical argumentation. Disability is a case in point. Ethicists have often taken for granted the association of disability with lesser well-being. From this starting point, bioethicists have discussed questions surrounding the termination of pregnancy, embryo selection and embryo editing. Even those ethicists who have argued against such technologies have often used arguments related to the sanctity of life or the riskiness of the procedures while not questioning the assumption of diminished well-being. In her paper *Epistemic Oppression and Ableism in Bioethics*, Christine Wieseler states, 'Philosophers of disability have argued that disabled people face, due to ableism, testimonial and hermeneutical injustice — two forms of epistemic injustice — within the discourse of bioethics as well as within the practice of medicine' (Wieseler, 2020). Indeed, testimonial injustice, as described by Miranda Fricker in her book *Epistemic Injustice*, is the injustice that specific knowers are subjected to when they are ignored in their capacity as knowers because of certain stereotypes that prevail about such knowers (Fricker, 2009). A case in point is some autism researchers' reluctance to take testimonials of autistic people about empathy seriously because they would lack sufficient insight into their own emotions. This is a missed opportunity for autism researchers and a form of injustice. Hermeneutical injustice is the injustice suffered by those who think their experiences are not shared by others. Therefore, they consider their own experiences as idiosyncratic and not worthy of broader attention. This may happen, for example, if the words are lacking to describe specific experiences. Fricker gives the example of a woman in the fifties of the twentieth century who suffers from sexual harassment in the workplace. Given that these experiences were not often shared at that time, she may feel that she is alone, that this is normal or that she has no recourse.

Wieseler adds several other types of epistemic oppression, wilful hermeneutical ignorance, epistemic exploitation, and epistemic imperialism, that should pause bioethicists. Wilful hermeneutical ignorance is a term first described by Gaile Polhaus. It represents cases where marginalized groups explicitly make sense of their experiences but are ignored. It is the 'refusal of dominantly situated knowers to allow a warranted revision to shared hermeneutical resources' (Wieseler, 2020). For example, I remember a reproductive ethics discussion with a clinician on the termination of pregnancy in the case of a disability. The clinician considered the fact that parents of disabled children often state that they cherish their lives with their children and are happy as a form of cognitive dissonance. Disregarding disabled people's testimonials about their well-being for the same reason is also a form of wilful hermeneutical ignorance. It is a form of epistemic oppression or exclusion. Even if marginalized groups are asked to share their experience for science and policymakers to benefit from, this often takes the form of epistemic exploitation. People are asked to spend time and energy contributing to research endeavours without payment or being recognized as possessing equally important knowledge. It is still up to the researchers to decide which parts of the shared knowledge they will use. They sometimes do not revise their underlying assumptions even after correction by those with experiential knowledge. It is an experience that many autistic people have had when contributing to research. They are invited to join advisory boards in autism research projects to give feedback. In the end, the research continues with the same premises and goals as before, without taking the input from the autistic community seriously. Hence, epistemic exploitation legitimises the epistemic agency of dominantly situated knowers. It is a form of window dressing.

Epistemic oppression causes rifts between scientists and the subjects they are studying and is a huge missed opportunity for developing scientific practices that are theoretically sound and that matter. It can be a requirement of the job of the bioethicist to ensure that clinical research projects engage those with unique knowledge and experience from the moment a project proposal is written. We should also advocate for more acknowledgement of the time and effort spent and urge funding agencies to set aside money for the engagement of different stakeholders. Wieseler also describes epistemic imperialism, another phenomenon that entrenches the epistemic agency of dominantly situated knowers. It refers to forcing the dominant belief systems on oppressed groups by suggesting that these systems are value-free or 'just the way it is'. Such imperialism needs not to be intentional. Even practices of inclusion may be imperialist. Wieseler states that 'bioethicists purport to make objective epistemic claims that are actually informed by ableist hermeneutical resources' (Wieseler, 2020). We may be as inclusive as we like: If we do not question our ableist take on issues relating to well-being and quality of life, this is still a form of epistemic imperialism. The opposite is true: non-disabled bioethicists are disadvantaged in knowing about disability and quality of life. If, for instance, the dominant position in reproductive ethics is the assumption that a disabled person's life will be worse or less joyful than the life of a non-disabled person, it would effectively underlie discussions over who gets to live. Therefore not questioning one's prejudices has far-reaching repercussions.

I think we can learn from standpoint theory that we must take the situated knowledge of those who are disabled seriously. This will yield different philosophical and ethical knowledge, improving the stance we often take for granted. It is, moreover, also a question of justice. I believe that bioethics, bearing in mind what is at stake in the conclusions we draw, should engage actively with the literature on epistemic standpoints and injustice and urge researchers, research consortia and research funders to take these ideas seriously. That does not mean that striving for epistemic justice and engaging situated knowledge is not without its challenges. In some respects, standpoint epistemology is still somewhat intellectualistic. It is not merely using empirical research methods such as surveys and qualitative research to discover other people's experiences, values, and norms. There is no guarantee that participants of marginalized groups do not reproduce the dominant discourse. Therefore, an approach based on the insights from standpoint epistemology should be more than a representation of opinions. It is actively thinking about the situatedness of your knowledge. Thus, it is quite demanding from the groups whose views it tries to incorporate. Nevertheless, if we take the idea of situated knowledge seriously, it means that the knowledge of those who typically are not represented should be considered. Even more so than physical disability, there is a dearth of knowledge about the experiences of those who do not have a voice, either because they do not communicate with oral speech, like some autistic people, or because they have an intellectual disability that prevents them from participating in a specific discourse. I believe that also here, the bioethicist can play a role.

The Role of the Bioethicist: Diplomats and Idiots

In March 2020, I got COVID-19. Although I considered it mild at the time, as I did not end up in the hospital, I had cognitive issues and extreme tiredness for months afterwards. Even upon writing these words, my pre-pandemic energy levels are still not back, and neither is my sense of smell fully restored. Such is life. However, in the months after that first wave, many people started to have similar experiences, sometimes far more debilitating than mine. The phenomenon became known as long COVID-19 and has been considered an actual phenomenon, an actual disease, despite initial hesitance to take these symptoms seriously as more than post-infection fatigue or pandemic anxiety. This recognition came about thanks to the patient organizations that arose in the aftermath of the first couple of waves. Although I was, and am still, very reluctant to talk about my health situation, I did talk a bit about long COVID-19, and I became known as someone with the symptoms.

At the same time, I am also a professor, an academic bioethicist. Because of that double role, I was invited to talk about my symptoms at a symposium by and for medical professionals. I was in the grey zone, being both someone with experience and an academic. The organizers were reluctant to invite representatives of patient organizations, presumably because they wanted to hear what they considered a more 'neutral' voice. My academic credits gave me an entrance ticket. This experience gave me pause: after all, I was there to talk about my experiences, not about my academic work. On the one hand, I thought it was self-evident that a patient representative has relevant experience. Their experience may be less tainted with conceptual and ethical flutter. On the other hand, maybe I was in a position to argue for the stakeholder precisely because of my specific situation, having a double identity as a patient and as a bioethicist. I had credibility in both ways. I have advocated for incorporating the autistic experience in autism research and have gained some credibility among autism researchers. However, I do not have a diagnosis of autism myself, making me an outsider both among autism researchers and autistic people. At the same time, it seems unfair that all the burden of giving credibility to experiences should go to those with the experiences. Autistic researchers, for one, sometimes just want to be seen as researchers, not as spokespersons. I believe that there is an essential role for the bioethicist to play. As intermediaries between research and experience, we can make medicine more just and truthful, which are not necessarily separate endeavours. During the long COVID-19 symposium, some clinicians were reluctant to accept the phenomena described by patients as accurate. A neurologist stressed that neurological and psychological tests are needed to objectify the long

COVID-19 experiences. They may have had a point that it is essential to link experiences to what we know already. However, we may miss important information if this is used to add credibility to experiences. Existing 'objective' tests can only investigate what is already known. In the case of long COVID-19, some of the cognitive symptoms that people describe are new and hard to catch in tests, such as the sudden loss of words to describe familiar things. Unless we take people's accounts for granted, we may never find 'objective' ways to test this. In what follows, I want to think about the bioethicist's role in clinical research some more. Specifically, I will argue that it is also our task to function as diplomats, in the words of Isabelle Stengers (Stengers, 2005). We are at home in the grey zone between science and the people experiencing what is researched. Especially in cases where people are reluctant or unable to convey their messages, we have to find ways to step in.

The role of bioethicists has been described as 'the handmaidens of medicine'. Bioethicists working with scientists on extensive research projects are often engaged to 'do' the obligatory ethics part. Mainly such work includes dealing with consent forms and interviewing stakeholders and the general public about their opinions regarding the matter. They are often asked to participate in the final weeks before the project's deadline. In the first part of this book, I argued that the role of philosophers and ethicists is at the heart of a research project, from the beginning to the end, querying implications and helping researchers get the concepts and aims of a project right. In other words, as they are trained to analyse ideas, assumptions, and implications, ethicists are best suited to be 'benevolent gadflies' in different types of research. However, being an ethicist on a research project also entails ensuring that the voices and interests of those directly affected by the project are heard. This is especially true if they are unable to raise their voices themselves. Isabelle Stengers's idea of the diplomat, as she describes it in her article *The cosmopolitical proposal*, can inspire this position (Stengers, 2005). In this paper, she urges us to '"slow down" reasoning and create an opportunity to arouse a slightly different awareness of the problems and the situations mobilizing us'. She uses the word cosmopolitical and not cosmopolitan on purpose. For her, it is not about attaining a final world order we would consider 'good' for everyone, as in Kant's idea of citizenship. Instead, for her, cosmos refers to 'the unknown constituted by these multiple, divergent worlds, and to the articulations of which they could eventually be capable, as opposed to the temptations of a peace intended to be final, ecumenical'.

Particularly inspiring is Stengers' reference to Deleuze's *idiot*, a concept that Deleuze himself borrowed from Fyodor Dostoevsky. This idiot 'is the one who always slows the others down, who resists the consensual way in which the situation is presented and in which emergencies mobilize thought or actions'. As bioethicists, we can be such idiots operating in the grey zone. I confess that I have also played the idiot's role in autism research projects, asking questions that annoy more serious scientists. Such questions included: What does it mean that your project will help autistic children? What does helping autistic children mean? What does autistic mean? And so on. I do not think I am an annoying person per se, but I believe that such interventions enable different viewpoints, angles, and alternative views. Maybe such a task is at the heart of the role of the bioethicist or the philosopher of science, to take nothing for granted, to sow seeds of hesitation or potentially new ways of approaching phenomena. I would thus argue that bioethicists be such *idiots*.

Besides idiots, we can also be diplomats. The role of the diplomat is, according to Stengers,

> to give a voice to those who define themselves as threatened, in a way likely to cause the experts to have second thoughts, and to force them to think about the possibility that their favourite course of action may be an act of war. (Stengers, 2005)

For those who cannot or do not want to speak for themselves,

> witnesses can make them present, conveying what it may feel like to be threatened by an issue that one has nothing to contribute to.

If we want to take the ethics of bioethics seriously, we must take up that role, which is partly a political role. It means looking out for those who fall outside a utilitarian calculus, for those who are considered expendable. Bioethics has sometimes fallen into the trap of aiming for the 'utopian' vision of science and politics that Stengers describes and resists. An example that immediately springs to mind is the thought experiment used in reproductive genetics. It asks us to imagine a future where you have to fill out, on paper, the characteristics that your future child would have. The argument goes that we will end up in a society without disabilities. Although many bioethicists would grant that disabled people often do live a worthwhile and happy life, the idea is that all things considered, a society without disabilities is better than one with disability. In that respect, there are no real arguments against not wishing for disability. However, as we will see in Part Four, such utopian projects are misguided, as they try to abstract from the messiness of the world, from the fact that there are many divergent worlds that all have a claim to what is well-being—the good life—one no less valid than the other. There is no answer to whether a world without disability is better than a world with disability: the question itself is nonsensical. There is no vantage point on which we could stand and from which we can apply our general principle of a good life, separate from the diverse people that live their lives. Instead, a more helpful role for ethicists is that of a witness for those who are not heard or the diplomat for those whose interests or experiences tend to be neglected. Stengers states that:

> As for the cosmopolitical perspective, its question is twofold. How to design the political scene in a way that actively protects it from the fiction that 'humans of good will decide in the name of the general interests'? How to turn the virus or the river into a cause for thinking? But also how to design it in such a way that collective thinking has to proceed in the presence of 'those who would otherwise be likely to be disqualified as having idiotically nothing to propose, hindering the emergent' common account. (Stengers, 2005)

I believe that the bioethicist can play various roles here, for example, as part of a consortium on vaccination strategies during pandemics. Alternatively, as part of an evaluation panel deciding on project funding for research that aims to 'treat' autism. Or perhaps as part of a working group devising new strategies to tackle biodiversity loss. Our task is to make things more complex rather than strip questions of their complexity and to resist science and ethics that neglect complexity.

PART FOUR
TROUBLES

In which I give four suggestions to build a framework for an ethics of life

Philosophically and materially, I am a compostist, not a posthumanist. Beings — human and not — become with each other, compose and decompose each other, in every scale and register of time and stuff in sympoietic tangling, in earthly worlding and unworlding. All of us must become more ontologically inventive and sensible within the bumptious holobiome that Earth turns out to be, whether called Gaia or a Thousand Other Names.

– Donna Haraway

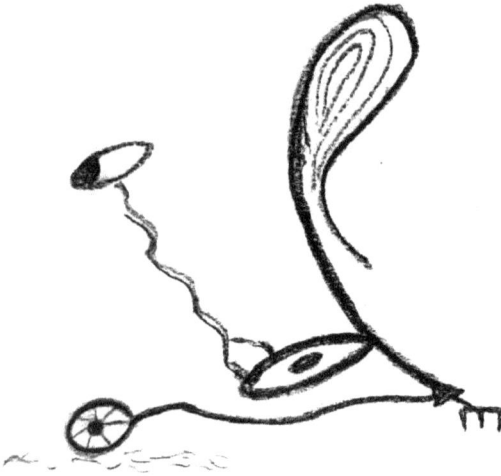

Cool Warm Lady.

How to reveal the hidden beast of burden of fellow sapiens?

From: Direct intuitive capturing of the hidden beast of burden accompanying a woman in the tram.

Sketch by Bartaku, 2018[1]

---

1   Beast of Burden series: practice of enhancing attunement. Bartaku Art_Research (unpublished).

In the previous three parts, I sketched what I believe to be an acceptable ontology and epistemology for the ethics of life in all its aspects. In Part One, I gave a view of science based on a developmental view of organisms. In Part Two, I sketched what ideas from process philosophy can mean for bioethics. In Part Three, I described how such a view of life as constantly developing, finding new ways, and engaging with chance encounters, also applies to pathology. Studying and understanding life, health and pathology means leaving behind ivory towers and 'God tricks'. It means acknowledging that knowledge is situated and evolving and that the knowledge we generate will yield different situations to think with. At the same time, large-scale events such as the COVID-19 pandemic and nuclear threats from Russia's invasion of Ukraine urge us to reconsider our relationship with the environment and the future. Bioethics that focuses on particular experiences, on global and even existential dangers, does not have to be a contradiction.

In this chapter, I suggest the foundations on which bioethics for the future could rest. I recapitulate the basic ideas of the previous chapters and explain how they can guide the bioethicist in everyday work, using different cases. First, I discuss the necessity and challenges of a rapprochement between environmental and medical ethics. Second, I present care ethics as a moral theory to guide all ethical theories. Third, I argue the need to appreciate the context sensitivity of specific challenges and engage with existing injustices. Fourth, I point out that creative engagement with the humanities can help develop stories for a liveable future.

13. Bringing Back the Environment

In Part Three, I advocated reassessing how traditional bioethics has dealt with disability. In thought experiments and policy decisions, disability is too often thought of as inevitably linked with burden and suffering. I have suggested an approach that incorporates, and perhaps even starts from, idiosyncratic life experience and acknowledges that all scientific and bioethic thought is built upon a foundation of pre-existing and contextual knowledge. It may appear that thinking about disability is mainly relevant to medical ethics; in thinking about health and disease. However, disability may also shed a different light on our *environmental* responsibility. Recall that Van Rensselaer Potter dreamed of a single discipline which integrated medical and environmental ethics. In Part One, I sketched how a developmental, epigenetic way of thinking about organisms suggests an intricate entanglement between organisms and the environment. Indeed, scholars such as Josep Santaló and María Berdasco have argued that epigenetics may provide a bridge between biomedical ethics and environmental ethics (Santaló and Berdasco, 2022). In Part Three, Canguilhem's approach sheds a different light on how we think of pathology. 'Life is experience', according to Canguilhem, and understanding life and the ethics of life entails understanding experience—our own experience and that of other creatures. That health and environment are intricately linked needs no further proof.

At the time of writing this book, we are in the second year of the COVID-19 pandemic, a pandemic linked to biodiversity loss. Bioethicists are also considering the relevance of the environment for health and medical ethics. For example, Cristina Richie has pointed out that bioethicists engage with environmental policies in two ways (Richie, 2019). On the one hand, the impact of health technologies and medicine on the environment can be part of an ethical deliberation on new technologies and treatments. The pandemic has demonstrated the

 https://doi.org/10.11647/OBP.0320.13

effects of the enormous amount of disposable mouth masks and home tests produced for all of us. Both items were probably essential to battle the pandemic, but we can only start to imagine the excessive amount of waste they generate. On the other hand, there is the impact of climate change and environmental damage, such as pollution, on our health. Since the turn of the century and the advent of genomic technologies, personalised and precision medicine have heralded a new paradigm in medicine, so it seems. This evolution has not escaped bioethicists: the vast amount of personal data has generated challenges concerning privacy and solidarity with researchers. The main goal of preventive or personalised medicine seems to be preventing rather than curing diseases. Precision medicine hopes to offer personalised recommendations based on biomarkers. With these recommendations, people can take their health into their own hands and adjust their lifestyles. In light of current and future pandemics and the nuclear threat in 2022, we may wonder whether this emphasis on personal responsibility, under the guise of personal empowerment, is not misguided. Surely the advice to eat healthier or get more physical exercise is, although sound, leading us away from the significant threats to our health related to climate change and pollution?

Potter argued for bioethics that is essentially forward-looking. Such bioethics values life and strives for the survival of life in general and humanity in particular. It encompasses personal health-related ethical questions and questions regarding the survival of humanity at large. He wrote his first book when Rachel Carson had described the devastating consequences of pesticide pollution in her book *Silent Spring* (Carson, 2002). At that point, it became more and more apparent that human beings are responsible for and have the power to alter their destiny — either survival or extinction. I appreciate this forward-looking aspect of his approach to bioethics. Given the times we are in, it makes sense to focus primarily on the survival of humankind and their kin, both in ethics and science. Moreover, we must make sure that this is not mere survival. Movies such as *Interstellar* have depicted humanity as worthy of saving no matter what, even if it means repopulating dire planets with what is left over from humanity. This is not my take. The ultimate goal is not survival per se but a livable future filled with joy and with what is valuable. It is a future that allows life in all its forms to continue creatively, seeking new possibilities based on chance encounters. Hence, imagining what kind of future we want to preserve is included within global bioethics. It means being informed by different types of living and reassessing our emphasis on cold rationality. It also means staying with the trouble of irreconcilable paradoxes and accepting failures from which we can learn. However, before we get there, I will describe what could be such a paradox with thinking about our responsibility to future generations.

I have described how thought experiments in bioethics often ask us to imagine a future without disability. Such thought experiments ask us to choose between a future with and a future without disability and then argue that everyone in their right mind would choose a future without, especially if we assume that the future is as bleak as forecasts tell us. If we look at mainstream contemporary apocalyptic fiction, both in games, films, and literature, in post-apocalyptic survival mode, it is those with disabilities that draw the shortest straw. Such an image aligns with crude interpretations of Darwin's survival of the fittest. People often assume it corresponds to how life would have been in the early days of humanity when we were cave dwellers in a harsh world or started to become farmers, and optimal productivity became the prime directive. However, this is neither the only possible past nor the only possible future. In their monumental book *The Dawn of Everything*, David Graeber and David Wengrow describe Romito 2, a 10,000-year-old burial site in which the remains of a male with a rare genetic disorder were found (Graeber and Wengrow, 2021). In life, the male had acromesomelic dysplasia — a condition affecting the growth of the bones in the forearms and legs. This story offers an antidote to the perception that disability had no place in human prehistory. In the same way, post-apocalyptic and speculative fiction may depict a future in which caring for each other gives meaning to survival.

Still, there may be another paradox left to deal with when it comes to disability, the environment, and the prevention of disability. How can we consider environmental factors that cause disability as *bad* but disability in itself as value-neutral? Some reproductive ethicists argue in favour of termination in the case of pregnancy if the child will be born with a disability. Pregnant people are urged to refrain from smoking and alcohol to avoid disability in their future offspring. When we go to such lengths to prevent disability, why don't we consider disability in itself as bad? How to respect the views of disabled people who want to be cured? Thomas H. Bretz tackles the point of tension between environmental justice and disability advocacy in their paper *Discussing Harm without Harming: Disability and Environmental Justice.* (Bretz, 2020) They write,

> This tension arises from the fact that environmental justice literature and media coverage usually portray disability as an automatic harm that must be avoided. Contrariwise, most disability study's authors and activists reject this view and suggest we 'understand... a sustainable world as a world that has disability in it'.

A similar feeling is described by Eli Clare in their book *Brilliant Imperfection, Grappling with Cure* (Clare, 2017). They wonder how we can appreciate bodies in all their forms, including disabled ones, and at the same time condemn the environmental pollution that has caused them:

> Amidst this cacophony, you want to know how to express your hatred of military pollution without feeding the assumption that your body-mind is tragic, wrong, and unnatural. No easy answers exist. You and I talk intensely; both the emotions and the ideas are dense. We arrive at a slogan for you: 'I hate the military and love my body.'
>
> Undoubtedly we could have come up with a catchier or more complex slogan. Nonetheless, it lays bare an essential question: how do we witness, name, and resist the injustices that reshape and damage all kinds of body-minds — plant and animal, organic and inorganic, nonhuman and human — while not equating disability with injustice? (Clare, 2017, p. 56)

Bretz suggests a way out of the dilemma. They argue that disabled persons suffer the most from environmental insults and other health hazards. The impact of pollution on people with asthma is a case in point. The COVID-19 pandemic, which could be considered an environmental hazard, has illustrated the impact on disabled people, as they were often affected the most by an infection. Bretz refers to Elizabeth Barnes, who points out a normative difference between being disabled and becoming disabled (Barnes, 2016). Barnes considers the first a neutral state (the mere difference view, as she calls it), whereas the latter involves shifting from one form of embodiment to another. Hence, Bretz suggests, we must separate environmental injustice from persons, irrespective of how they are embodied (Barnes, 2016).

Bretz suggests an account of environmental wrongdoing that does not rely on ableist assumptions about being disabled. Instead, Bretz uses Barnes's mere difference view to show that disability in itself is neutral. Nevertheless, that does not imply that there cannot be harm associated with disability for specific people. However, these harms are always context-dependent and go hand in hand with environmental or psychological factors. How can we then still argue in favour of environmental justice? Bretz suggests that we should still look at the change in disability rates in a particular environment as a reason for an investigation into environmental hazards. If we find these toxic environments, we can object to them because they may have problematic effects, such as the death of organisms, illnesses, or structural damage to DNA. Of course, here we hit a limitation of Bretz's approach: we can assume that death is bad, but the dividing line between illnesses, structural DNA damage, and disability is hard to draw. When does something become harmful and not a neutral difference?

Bretz also argues that we can look at the process rather than the outcome: if your embodiment is changed against your will, either from disabled to non-disabled and vice versa, this is wrong not because the procedure is bad, per se, but because there was no consent given. Moreover, we can examine whether harmful facilities and structures have been established following democratic deliberation. Bretz argues that, at the same time, we shouldn't deny that disability can involve harm for some in combination with other factors. A specific type of embodiment can be less optimal in certain contexts. We are reminded of Georges Canguilhem. Moreover, we can consider the particular way pollution induces these changes as harmful. Pollution interferes with people's bodies without their consent. Hence, Bretz states that the normative evaluation is of the trespass, not the embodiment.

I appreciate Bretz's approach, which helps us understand environmental justice and disability justice as entangled. However, it seems impossible to make an argument that is watertight in all aspects. For example, what about toxic insults on embryos? Or on the primordial stem cells of men before they become fathers? These insults will affect any offspring that are potentially conceived years later. Bretz acknowledges this and states that, in this case, consent for environmentally-induced changes in embodiment at early developmental stages is either unreasonable to assume (foetus), impossible (the affected person) or very unlikely (the pregnant person).

Embodiment is also tightly linked to one's identity, and we are hitting the identity problem hard here. Environmental insults that affect a person's embodiment before or even right after they are conceived probably are identity affecting, in that the person that develops from the embryo that has experienced the insult will be different from the person that would have developed without the environmental insult. How do you object to something that has made you as you are? In this way, such prenatal events may be more identity-affecting than when a different embodiment results from an injury or surgery. Bretz gives good reasons and strategies for environmental justice that avoids ableist arguments. However, maybe, in the end, Eli Clare's paradox, loving your body but hating the military that has caused it to be as it is, seems unresolved.

Perhaps the apparent incompatibility of these two thoughts is not as problematic as it seems at first sight. The desire to dissolve paradoxes is, I think, related to a tendency in Western ethics to want ethics to be rational and consistent at all times. To a certain extent, ethical reflections have to be rational. Nevertheless, at the same time, ethics is not a waterproof system, nor does it need to be. Maybe the example of disability and the environment teaches us two things. Fighting environmental pollution, appreciating different ways of embodiment, and fighting ableist assumptions in the fight for environmental justice are all essential moral imperatives that can stand on their own. It may be impossible to bring them together in a grand watertight scheme. That does not mean that the incompatibility of our different values should be fatalistically accepted. Nor is this an argument that strengthens the idea that environmental and biomedical ethics are worlds apart. Paradoxes and incompatibilities have significant heuristic value: they teach us something about what is important. Such issues should be confronted head-on, not because we want to dissolve them, but because staying and thinking with the trouble of these inconsistencies may shed new light on what we value and what future we should imagine. This is, for example, a future without artificial pollution but one that simultaneously celebrates different ways of being embodied in the world. The case of disability offers a good starting point for forward-looking ethics.

Rosemarie Garland-Thomson calls disability 'the transformation of flesh as it encounters the world' (Garland-Thomson, 2012). Garland-Thomson writes that 'we will all become disabled if we live long enough and every life, every family has disability in it at some time' (Garland-Thomson, 2012). This acknowledgement of the omnipresence of disability is a fact that I believe many have forgotten when they have argued for specific policies during the pandemic. Thinking with disability, however, means imagining a future that can sustain all different types of embodiment. It requires an approach to bioethics beyond conventional principlist, utilitarian or deontological approaches, as these too often assume that ethics can be made watertight. In the next part, I will continue imagining what this approach could be like.

14. Caring Responsibilities

For those who make a living by talking and writing about ethics, it is often easy to forget that ethics never came in flavours of deontology or consequentialism; the principles of justice and autonomy and utility are not intrinsic properties of ethical problems. When we speak of ethical principles-or more fashionably, of a communitarian or a narrative ethic — we do so because we find these useful ways of thinking about ethics: as a self-standing conceptual system by which we can impose some sort of order upon ethical questions. But in reality, ethics does not stand apart. It is one thread in the fabric of society and it is intertwined with others. Ethical concepts are tied to a society's customs, manners, traditions, institutions- all of the concepts that structure and informs the ways that a member of that society deals with the world. When we forget this, we are in danger of leaving the world of genuine moral experience for the world of moral fiction, a simplified, hypothetical creation suited less for practical difficulties than for intellectual convenience.

– Carl Elliott, *A Philosophical Disease* (Elliott, 1999, p. 146)

In a thought-provoking reflection on bioethics, *A Philosophical Disease*, Carl Elliott challenges the traditional toolkit of the bioethicist (Elliott, 1999). This toolkit consists of moral theories such as consequentialism, deontology, and principles. Elliott argues that they are not sufficient to deal with the complexity and even messiness of the actual world, nor should ethics be seen as an all-encompassing system that guides everything from the outside. I ended the previous chapter with the idea that it is best to stay with the trouble of accepting that ethical reflection is and always will be partial and messy—at least in the case of the seeming incompatibility of disability discourse and arguing against environmental pollution. At the same time, bioethics is *practical* ethics: we are often asked to develop concrete recommendations and ways to go forward with a specific new biomedical technology. The principles and moral theories we have been educated with and which we use to educate

https://doi.org/10.11647/OBP.0320.14

our students help clarify arguments and help us see the weaknesses and inconsistencies in our argumentations. Acknowledging the situatedness of ethical knowledge and the incompatibility of specific values does not mean that we have to give up on searching for clarity, nor that relativism— or even defeatism—is our only option. The existing bioethics toolkit can be of great assistance there. Perhaps the bioethical principles were never meant to answer ethical questions straightforwardly. Considering the context, circumstances, and particularities of specific ethical dilemmas are components of the practice of (bio)ethics, specifically in medical ethics.

The traditional bioethics approach has its limitations. A case in point is the rights of parents and their children. Children pose a significant challenge to conventional approaches to bioethics. They are gradually acquiring autonomy, one of the chief principles of bioethics. Hence, as long as they are not fully autonomous beings who can consent to their healthcare, principles such as beneficence and non-maleficence seems to trump respecting their autonomy. It remains uncertain to what extent and at which point the child's autonomy should be respected more than the parent's autonomy to decide on the best course of action for their child. The case of ADHD medication in children illustrates this. If a twelve-year-old wants to stop taking their medication, but the parents insist, what is the 'good' here? In medicine, it is often presumed that parents want the best for their children and have an ultimate say. But this need not always be the case, and parents may be wrong in some respects regarding the decisions they make for their children, or children may disagree with the decisions parents make. The child can also be wrong, but educating children always assumes some leeway for them to be misguided. After all, learning to fail is part of growing up. Dissecting parents' and children's potentially conflicting rights and duties using our traditional conceptual toolkit and ethical principles can be helpful. Such an approach can point out inconsistencies and gaps in knowledge. It can help clarify our thoughts about the matter and demonstrate where we need more empirical knowledge. For example, if we ask ourselves what authority parents have over their children and at which point children can have a say about their healthcare, we must acknowledge that this is highly dependent on culture and family tradition. It seems wrong and unnecessary to impose a standard 'from above' regarding the moment children have autonomy, and their parents' judgment does not count. At the same time, having a general principle that the autonomy of children is important can make explicit certain unethical situations more quickly. Children are nodes in a relational network, and it is artificial to think about their autonomy rights as separate from that network. Still, autonomy rights matter too. By prying apart the respective interests of children and parents in the first move, we can bring them together better in the second move. It seems what matters is a general acknowledgement of the importance of care and relations as a foundation from which to think about the rights and duties of parents and children. In its simplest form, caring can refer to parents' care towards their children, but it also means caring for children's growing independence and caring for parents in complex choices. Care is not trivial. Applying principles such as autonomy and beneficence may help point out inconsistencies in conventional moral thinking, resulting in actual changes. However, principles are just that: tools that help thinking and help shed some light on different aspects that matter. Besides these tools, we need a common ground for action that is grounded in how the world works and serves as a beacon for forward-looking ethics for a liveable future. I think a care ethics approach can offer such guidance.

In Western philosophy, care ethics is a relatively modern idea. It originates from Carol Gilligan's well-known critique of Kohlberg's stages of morality (Gilligan, 1982). When writing *Global Bioethics*, Potter acknowledged the advantages of feminist approaches to morality, such as Gilligan's.

> The global bioethic must be based on a combination of rights and responsibilities in which masculinity and femininity are no longer viewed as mutually exclusive dimensions of a bipolar continuum. The concept of psychological androgyny, the endorsing of certain traditional attitudes of both males and females, and the rejection of certain others, can reorganise traditional perspectives on sex roles. The greatest barrier to the widespread acceptance of a global bioethic is the 'macho' morality of male autonomy and dominance: dominance over women, with unlimited reproductive function in males, and confinement of women to the reproductive role; dominance over nature; and conflict with other males. This macho morality is in part the source for the belief that a technological fix can be found for any technological disaster and for the belief that religious Holy Wars are manly. In contrast, perhaps the greatest hope for acceptance of a global bioethic is the women's movement

for reproductive freedom, followed by the 'changed understanding of human development and a more generative view of human life' as imagined by Gilligan. (Potter, 1988, p. 90)

Given its strong emphasis on relationality and the particularities of personal relations, care ethics is also popular among feminist bioethicists (Lindemann, 2006). At the same time, care ethics has been vetted against other approaches to bioethics, for example, principlist approaches that stress autonomy or other principles. Precisely because of this, it is sometimes claimed that in medical encounters, an ethics of care can clash with an individual's right to autonomy. For example, a caring nurse may object to the wish of a palliative patient for euthanasia. However, it is also possible to consider respect for autonomy an integral part of care. Care ethics stresses relationality, and we can also look at the right to decide for ourselves from that relational perspective. For example, a caring approach to respect for autonomy in the case of euthanasia means thinking with the person requesting this, making them feel they are not alone in their decision. It may also imply caring for and understanding the doubts and feelings of those surrounding them. It is based on a view of life that stresses partnership and embodied communication, paraphrasing philosopher Eva Kittay (Kittay, 2019). It is, therefore, never one-directional. We are all interdependent and in need of care. Care, according to Kittay, is an ongoing process: it helps the one receiving care flourish, but they must implicitly or explicitly endorse the care offered (Skarsaune, Hanisch and Gjermestad, 2021). An ethics of care should also be seen as more than virtue ethics for doctors, nurses, and parents. Although some authors situate care firmly on the level of interpersonal relations between human beings, philosophers such as Joan Tronto have argued that an ethic of care should also have a political component. In the book *Caring Democracies*, Tronto defines caring as follows:

On the most general level, we suggest that caring be viewed as a species activity that includes everything that we do to maintain, continue and repair our 'world' so that we can live in it as well as possible. (Tronto, 2013, p. 19)

A bioethics that takes up a care ethic as its foundation is not a parochial endeavour that only 'cares about' interpersonal and private relationships. Bioethics should span both the individual and the political and consider how these are always intertwined. For starters, stressing the pervasive importance of caring for humans and other lives is in stark contrast with the attention paid to policymaking and economics. The pandemic has shown that jobs that involve caring are of utmost importance but are not traditionally linked with prestige or high wages. Care ethicists such as Joan Tronto have urged us to reconsider this and see concerns about real people's lives as an integral part of politics.

An ethic of care that is useful for bioethicists transcends the merely human and reflects an underlying truth that human existence is entangled with the world at large. Therefore, relationality is not only between human beings but between humans and different entities, from other-than-human animals to microbes and the environment. Indeed, in Maria Puig de la Bellacasa's ground-breaking work *Matters of Care*, she starts from Tronto's idea of care as a complex, life-sustaining web and describes care as intrinsically ethical and political (de la Bellacasa, 2017). Care thus transcends the often-believed between the ethical and political. Puig de la Bellacasa advocates a concept of posthuman care that transcends the mere inter-personal and inter-human. She describes care as 'a generalised condition that circulates through the stuff and surface of the world' (de la Bellacasa, 2017). Thus, care is a way to think about environmental and health ethics together. It reflects an underlying truth of human existence and our entanglement with the world at large, a truth that we also find in indigenous knowledge and ecofeminism.

Environmental ethics approaches often either take the flavour of anthropocentrism or ecocentrism. Anthropocentrism refers to the belief that value is human-centred and that all other beings are means to human ends. Environmental ethics often see it as the cause of our current environmental crises (Kopnina *et al.*, 2018). However, a more positive appreciation could be that, although anthropocentrism starts from the assumption that human beings are the primary concern, this can urge us to environmental action. If we value human life, taking environmental action is all the more important. Ecocentrism, in contrast, views human beings as an intrinsic part of nature and considers other life, and nature in itself, as having an intrinsic value. Arne Naess's deep ecology is an example of an ecocentric approach (Naess, 1986). I also consider myself on the side of ecocentrism. I think humankind's insistence on its superiority is misguided and even dangerous. At the same time, it is hard, and perhaps impossible, not to put one's human life and that of one's kin over that of other organisms. I think a care ethic approach to environmental ethics, such as we find in ecofeminism and indigenous approaches can show the way of thinking beyond the dualism of these two approaches. Vetting the rights of humans against the right of nature is not a fruitful approach. It must be possible to subscribe to an ontological ecocentrism and, at the same time, acknowledge the idea that specificity and entanglement with human and other-than-human others are morally relevant. From such a position, I think it is possible to take up an approach to environmental ethics that takes the ideas of care ethics at heart: it gives us grounds, and a method, for action. We are part of nature that has a value beyond us. However, we are also responsible for caring for nature so that we, and life in general, can recover and thrive (Cross, 2018). Acknowledging the entanglement of human well-being with environmental well-being demonstrates that environmental ethics and environmental justice are not separate things.

Such ideas are not new, nor is it very original thinking. Ecofeminists have been advocating these ideas for decades, and what is more, it has been an intricate part of indigenous thinking for centuries and even millennia.[1] As Kyle Powys Whyte and Chris Cuomo conclude in their book chapter 'Ethics of Caring in Environmental Ethics: Indigenous and Feminist Philosophies':

> Feminist and indigenous conceptions of care ethics offer a range of ideas and tools for environmental ethics, especially ones that are helpful of unearthing deep connections and moral commitment and for guiding environmental decision making. [...] The gendered, feminist, historical, and decolonial dimensions of care ethics and related approaches to environmental ethics provide rich ground for rethinking and reclaiming the nature and depth of diverse relationships as the very fabric of social and ecological being. (Whyte and Cuomo, 2016)

V. F. Cordova describes how Native American philosophy views humans as primarily social, connected, and belonging to a specific place. This belonging implies that they do not 'own' a place but must maintain

---

1   This does not mean that indigenous concepts of care are necessarily conservative, fixed or even atavistic. Think about the concept of *Buen Vivir*, which is an adaptation of indigenous thinking to present-day realities(Acosta, 2012).

it and have intimate knowledge about it. Belonging has relevance for environmental ethics and biodiversity. Cordova writes:

> The ecosystem of which he [Edward O. Wilson] speaks so eloquently is made up of interacting and interdependent communities. It is time to see that humans are part of the ecological web and that they too play a vital role-not as stewards over an inferior and mindless nature-but as a necessary part of a healthy and diverse system of life. (Cordova, 2007, p. 207)

Caring for nature is more tricky than the ethics of governing, ruling or stewarding nature. It is risking that the person, organism, or system we care for is unruly, resists, and does not conform to expectations. For bioethicists, it means encountering the challenges that other beings may pose to our firm beliefs. It means staying with the trouble of messy realities. This means accepting that we can fail and learn from this failure. Engaging in ethical argumentation is more of a learning process than finding the correct arguments that prove our point. It also means always keeping in mind what we do it for: to help ensure that those who come after us can still live a joyful and worthwhile life.

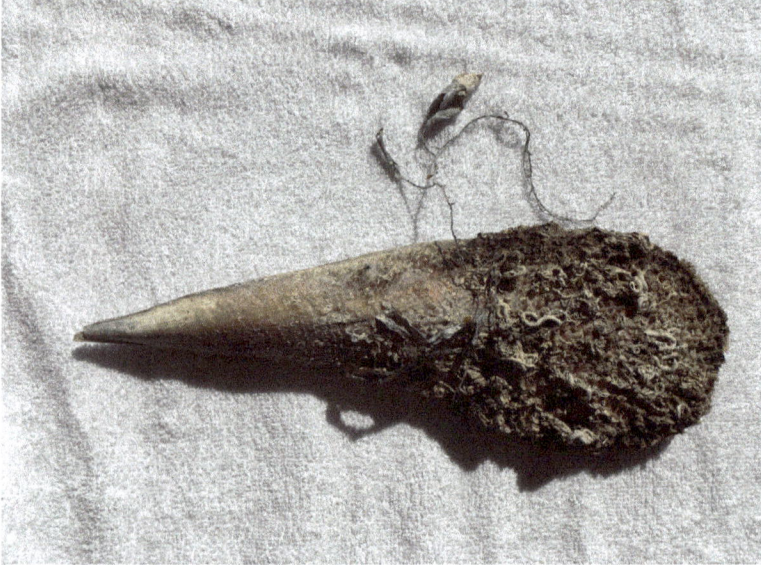

Untitled

How to be inclusive to companion species?

From: *Pinna Nobilis*, the Great Pen Shell, is the largest mollusc living in the Mediterranean Sea. Its intimate companion species are the Neptun Sea Grass (Posidonia oceanica) and other species that live on and inside the shell. Photo: Christina Stadlbauer, 2018[2]

---

2   The *Pinna nobilis* research was undertaken by the Institute for Relocation of Biodiversity in Sant'Antioco, Sardinia (Italy) and Mar Menor, South of Spain, between 2017–2019. The 40cm long shell on the photo was found in Mar Menor. They live in the shallow waters of the Mediterranean and in antiquity they were used for their byssus thread, a fine fibre that was crafted into sea-silk and used for decorative embroidery, https://christallinarox.wordpress.com/institute-for-relocation-of-biodiversity/

15. Unforgetting The Past

In urgent times, many of us are tempted to address trouble in terms of making an imagined future safe, of stopping something from happening that looms in the future, of clearing away the present and the past in order to make futures for coming generations. Staying with the trouble does not require such a relationship to times called the future. In fact, staying with the trouble requires learning to be truly present, not as a vanishing pivot between awful or Edenic pasts and apocalyptic or salvific futures, but as mortal critters entwined in myriad unfinished configurations of places, times, matters, meanings. Donna Haraway

— *Staying with the Trouble* (Haraway, 2016, p. 1)

In previous chapters, I have hinted at the idea that, given the existential predicaments we are facing, bioethics' prime directive must be a concern and care for a liveable future. At the same time, I have also stressed the need to incorporate standpoints and situated knowledge. For the first aspect, I am sympathetic to the project of Potter. The two books sketch bioethics that contributes to our species' survival. As we have seen in *Global Bioethics*, Potter mentions the importance of feminist perspectives and connects these with care and responsibility for the environment (Potter, 1988). However, because they neglect the importance of situated knowledge and learning from past experiences, these ideas cannot fully serve as a blueprint for 21st-century bioethics. For Potter, 'global bioethics' is grounded in biology. He thinks global bioethics yields values to which all cultures and religions can subscribe. These secular and universal values are 'quality of life' and 'quality of the environment', intricately interwoven. I agree that what makes life valuable is creativity, wisdom, joy, and a sense of belonging. In all of its specific cultural manifestations, this is linked to characteristics of life itself, and a 'good survival' is better than mere survival.

© 2022 Kristien Hens, CC BY-NC-ND 4.0   https://doi.org/10.11647/OBP.0320.15

Nevertheless, Van Rensselaer Potter does not seem to acknowledge that what constitutes 'quality of life' is also highly context and culture-specific. The emphasis on population control looks pretty US-centric and has little respect for the different roles that family values play in different cultures. Worse, Potter's suggestions are even colonial at specific points. For example, he mentions population growth in the Global South as something 'we' must tackle, and even the 'challenge of Islam to a global bioethics' (Potter, 1988). Such thoughts are unsupportable and dangerous and buy into a pro-Western sentiment that may be responsible for our current predicament in the first place.

On the contrary, starting from situated knowledge, bioethics should question its western-centric conception of good health and acknowledge that the concepts of good life and good health will vary. In the last chapter of *Global Bioethics*, Potter is genuinely visionary in that he describes the idea of 'personal health' and taking responsibility for one's health. He is a staunch advocate for what we would nowadays call preventive and precision medicine. He argues that people should take responsibility for their health by exercising, avoiding eating unhealthy foods, smoking, etc. Given his background in oncology, it is not difficult to see where the lists come from. At the same time, he seems to skim over and confuse systemic and personal causes and responsibilities. The 'personal health' of Potter or the personalised medicine paradigm of the 21st century is often anything but personal. It neglects lived experiences and cultural contexts in favour of a neutral idea of health. Moreover, it skims over existing inequalities and biases in health care in favour of stressing individual responsibilities for health.

Assuming that we have, or will be able to have, a society in which each takes up their responsibility equally is utopian. We can imagine taking a representative sample of Earth's organisms and terraforming a new world under a geodesic dome on Mars to solve the current environmental crisis. Such escapism is not a solution that forward-looking bioethics would suggest. As we have seen before, utopianism may look harmless and fun but often borders on totalitarianism and absolutist concepts of what kind of people should be there. Think about the thought experiment in which we are asked to imagine a future without disability. If we want forward-looking bioethics that imagines stories for humankind's survival and thriving, we must do so firmly anchored in the world as we know it and consider how it came about. Only then will we appreciate what kind of a future we can and may have.

We have seen how a process ontology such as Whitehead's suggests a world in flux in which our history and future are intimately connected. How do we creatively engage with the future while learning from the past? John Rawls sets out to think of an ideal theory we may design from behind a veil of ignorance. Rawls asks us to imagine that we do not know who we will become in the future (Rawls, 1999). Imagine that, from that starting position, we can start from scratch and invent a new society. If we do that, Rawls says, we cannot but think about society as one that offers equal opportunities for all. Rawls' thought experiment is a heartfelt plea for a more egalitarian society. For Rawls, such an ideal theory is what should guide us. Stuart Kauffman, whom we can also consider a process philosopher, critiques an ideal theory 'à la Rawls' that considers a clean slate solution to current inequalities:

> How we have struggled over this issue, because for given any claim to moral ought, we can ask, but is this moral ought really moral? On what ground? God? Kant's noumenal locus of 'moral ought'? Utilitarianism, 'the greatest good for the greatest number,' is unable to solve the problem of how justly to distribute the total 'good.' And morality and 'Justice' face further the fact that we do not always know the consequences. Rawls's (1971) post-Kantian efforts at Justice with his two rules: We behind a veil of ignorance in face of a society's institutions and would we choose them not knowing our station? And his effort at distribution: 'The most possible to the least of us.' But this is inadequate; our institutions evolve in ways we cannot say, including the US constitution where the Common Clause has been used for the drug war that has filled our prisons with too many black youths. We cannot design institutions; they grow, partly helter-skelter, with unintended consequences [...] No one time bargain, à la Rawls, will suffice. Our institutions, and we living in and through them, evolve in unprestatable ways. Are our ethics settled? Rawls likes the notion of 'reflective equilibrium.' But in the fourteenth century, the English practiced hanging, and drawing and quartering. Would we now? What is 'reflective equilibrium?' I doubt we ever come to reflective equilibrium. (Kauffman, 2016, p. 251)

Most bioethicists would agree with Kauffman that the exercise of reflective equilibrium does not yield a one-off conclusion. It must be constantly repeated. Today, many political philosophers question the possibility of such an ideal theory of justice. For example, in their paper on justice, Jenny Reardon and colleagues write:

> Justice is a powerful rhetoric that is itself hard to resist; thus, it can produce single-minded activism and a loss of criticality. These problems are compounded when justice is united with the universalisms of science. Much suffering has been wrought by hegemonic and colonial efforts to build universalized knowledge and justice together; a single knowledge and a single justice excludes too many. (Reardon *et al.*, 2015)

A non-ideal theory starts by considering existing injustices to narrate a liveable future. For example, Iris Marion Young has argued how structural injustices are closely related to historical injustices and how we have a collective responsibility to solve them as members of society (Young, 2011). Charles Mills has convincingly argued that approaches such as the one by Rawls neglect the racism on which current society is built (Mills and Mills, 1997). Bioethicists and political philosophy are traditionally separate disciplines, but bioethics has much to learn from non-ideal theory, as is demonstrated by the contributors of the volume *Applying Nonideal Theory to Bioethics: Living and Dying in a Nonideal World* (Victor and Guidry-Grimes, 2021). For example, we may be too quick in dreaming up, for example, a world without disability in our thought experiments. Such examples tend to ignore that the problem may not lie in disability's specific embodiment but in normalising and even oppressive tendencies.

In their book *An Intersectional Feminist Theory of Moral Responsibility*, Mich Ciurria paves the way to an intersectional feminist framework, with five central aims to evaluate existing inequalities and move forward from them (Ciurria, 2019). These aims are also applicable to bioethics. The first aim Ciurria has is foregrounding and diagnosing (especially systemic) intersections of injustice, oppression, and adversity. Indeed, forward-looking bioethics needs to be inspired by the voices of those who have traditionally not had a voice. For example, as bioethicists are often medical ethicists, they should be aware of biases and stereotypes that prevent people from minority groups from receiving adequate care. This first aim organically leads to the second aim: actively combating injustice, oppression and adversity. Indeed, by thinking about the future we want and being aware of current injustices, bioethicists are forced to vigorously fight these injustices and give a voice to those who traditionally did not have one. The third aim is to use an ameliorative method. This method goes beyond describing concepts to defining concepts by reference to ameliorative purposes, as Ciurria, following Sally Haslanger, describes. For example, bioethicists can, together with philosophers of medicine, consider concepts of health and pathology that start from the experiences and different embodiments of all kinds of people and acknowledge the impossibility of locating pathology solely in the individual. I think the ideas of Georges Canguilhem can inspire such an ameliorative approach. The fourth aim of an intersectional feminist approach, according to Ciurria, is the use of a relational method. They describe this as analysing existing relations of power and domination. If we apply this to bioethics, investigating the relationships of clinicians and researchers with patients and participants springs to mind. I think a relational method should not solely focus on power relations but also on empowering relations, on the possibility of all actors thinking with each other. The bioethicist's task is, then, to enable this thinking with. The fifth aim is to use a non-ideal theoretical method. With Ciurria, I believe ethics, and in this case, bioethics, must start from the messiness and injustices of the world. There is no place for naïve utopianism in this way of thinking. Instead, ethicists should think of themselves as the 'plumbers of philosophy' to speak with the words of Mary Midgley (Midgley, 1992). In sum, these five aims can help bioethicists stay with the trouble of past injustices and tell stories that incorporate future learning to make things better.

16. A Creative and Forward-Looking Bioethics

In the previous chapter, I described how, if we want to imagine and strive for a liveable future, a tabula rasa approach will not suffice. Instead, forward-looking bioethics should start from existing injustices and take an ameliorative approach. We saw in chapter two that Whitehead's process ontologies and Barad's new materialist ontologies include an essential aspect of world-making; creativity. Nevertheless, that does not mean that what is created is straightforwardly good. If wrong choices are made, creativity can lead to disaster. These ideas are close to V. F. Cordova's writing on *time* in *How it Is*:

> 'Indian time' is of a different sort. Since we are participants in a process of motion and change, we know that we can affect the future. If we chop down all the trees, we will live in a world without trees. If we have too many children, we will live in a state of overpopulation. There is no glorious 'future' out 'there' waiting for us to arrive. We build the future through our present actions. We do not, however, 'build' as gods but as participants in certain circumstances — not all events are of our own making. The universe is a process of which we are but a small part. (Cordova, 2007, pp. 119–120)

In the words of Donna Haraway, it matters what stories we tell. In the book *Meeting the Universe Halfway*, Karen Barad calls such an approach an 'ethico-onto-epistemology' (Barad, 2007). Barad describes an ethics of *mattering*. This ethics entails being accountable for the entanglements we help enact and the future we help create by every decision we make and every word we use. Such ethics is not ethics that is imposed from above, which uses moral theories and principles as their primary means. It is relational ethics, tightly linked to our materiality and being in the world. In a similar vein, Donna Haraway stresses the importance

https://doi.org/10.11647/OBP.0320.16

of *response-ability*. Haraway defines 'response-ability' as 'cultivating collective knowing and doing' (p. 34), 'sympoiesis' (making-with) (p. 58), and as responses of becoming-with and rendering each other capable. She writes:

> Hannah Arendt and Virginia Woolf both understood the high stakes of training the mind and imagination to go visiting, to venture off the beaten path to meet unexpected, non-natal kin, and to strike up conversations, to pose and respond to interesting questions, to propose together something unanticipated, to take up the unasked-for obligations of having met. (Haraway, 2016, p. 130)

It is thinking with each other and weaving together the stories we want to tell that will help us go forward with a liveable world. Thom Van Dooren expresses similar ideas in the introduction to the mesmerizing book *The Wake of Crows*, in which Van Dooren argues for multispecies ethics.

> In a context in which we all are, unavoidably, crafting worlds with others, multispecies ethics represents a commitment to worlding well, to contributing in whatever ways we can to the imagining and crafting of flourishing, abundant worlds. In Isabelle Stengers's terms, it is about 'accepting that what we add makes a difference in the world and becoming able to answer for the manner of this difference'. (Van Dooren, 2019, p. 14)

These are helpful ideas for bioethics, and they align with the path I have tried to pave. In the previous chapters, I argued for a care-full ethical practice, aiming for a liveable future and considering particular experiences and injustices. At the same time, it may not be straightforward to translate Barad's and Haraway's ideas into bioethical practice. Bioethicists practice applied ethics in different kinds of circumstances. They are required to help deal with dilemmas in clinical settings and more general questions about the desirability of novel technologies and questions of justice. Some work must be done to translate Barad's ethics of mattering or Donna Haraway's response-ability to bioethical practice. Still, I believe that their ideas are not that far removed from actual bioethical practice, although it seems like bioethicists and posthumanist thinkers often speak a different language. At the same time, bioethics has been concerned with individual values and contexts all along. Although it is often claimed that bioethics is an apolitical endeavour, most arguments in bioethics do touch upon or are relevant to policymaking. Different sensitivity to the stories we use and tell and the worlds we create through these stories can make the bioethical reflection more caring. A case in point may be the ethical questions that arose during the COVID-19 pandemic.

The COVID-19 pandemic was a wake-up call for bioethicists like me. Suddenly, it was assumed that we could prove our worth by thinking about the critical questions. We have been teaching trolley problems and survival lotteries for a long time, so now there was an opportunity to demonstrate that we can contribute to real-life discussions. Consider the question of who gets priority at the ICU if spaces are limited. Other examples are whether we can force people to be vaccinated: how to weigh people's right to decide for themselves with the duty to solidarity to get out of this situation as quickly as possible? However, such ad hoc disaster ethics, which may look like the only option at the moment, should not be the primary concern of bioethics. Donna Haraway and Maria Puig de la Bellacasa stress the importance of telling good stories which are capable of committing us to possible liveable worlds. Being response-able is not tackling ethical questions as they arrive. Nor is being response-able the same as buying into the utopianism in many bioethics thought experiments and 'what-ifs'. Often these include a sterile vision of the future in which disability, chance encounters, and complexity have no place. I believe that we need stories that help us stay with the trouble and, at the same time, work with the trouble to create a care-filled and relational world. Rather than thought experiments or sterile utopias, or dystopias, what is needed are real-life experiences and speculative fiction that does not explain away the messiness of the world. I am reminded of Rebecca Solnit's *Hope in the Dark* (Solnit, 2016). Solnit describes how we can be inspired by small victories in the past to find hope that there is still a future for humankind. For Solnit, hope is not an irrational belief that everything will be fine. She writes,

> To hope is to gamble. It's to bet on the future, on your desires, on the possibility that an open heart and uncertainty are better than gloom and safety. To hope is dangerous, and yet it is the opposite of fear, for to live is to risk. (Solnit, 2016, p. 4)

'Certainty', she writes, 'is despair. But it is *daring* to allow failure also in our moral judgements'. Referring to Native American origin stories and the character of the trickster coyote, she states: 'Coyote pisses on moral purity and rigid definitions'.

As the proverbial interdisciplinary meeting ground, bioethics can benefit from different methodologies. Bioethicists had undertaken empirical research in many various forms long before experimental philosophy became fashionable. Still, we can go further: besides the traditional qualitative and quantitative empirical methods, the importance of telling the correct stories hints at a rapprochement between bioethics and health humanities, and in fact, thinking these two together. For example, Maren Linett argues in the book *Literary Bioethics* that studying literary texts can significantly enhance our potential for a nuanced view of bioethical issues (Linett, 2020). I think Linett is right when she states that literature allows us bioethicists to venture outside our natural 'habitus'. Good literature will enable us to take 'imaginary leaps' and venture beyond our intuitive conceptions by confronting us with the thoughts and actions of rounded characters. Literature goes beyond the flattened narrative of a philosophical thought experiment and enables multiple readings. It unleashes the creative potential to unlock possible realities and truths. It does so regardless of the intention of the writer. For example, by presenting the thoughts and actions of characters with a cognitive disability, we are invited to revisit our preconceptions of what it means to lead a meaningful life. Linett gives the example of Kazuo Ishiguro's *Never Let Me Go* to investigate what it means to be human and worthy of (ethical) consideration. The presentation of human clones who are the same (if not fitter) as other humans make us reflect on the dividing line between who bears rights and who does not. It also makes us reflect on the arbitrary dividing line between the human and the other-than-human: *Never Let Me Go*'s protagonists are 'humanely' treated in a boarding school that enables them to develop their artistic and intellectual talents. Still, they are clones created explicitly so that their organs can be harvested once they are in their twenties. Linett argues that Ishiguro's book can be read as a commentary on humane farming: the idea that, at least for other-than-human animals (or for clones), death in itself is not a bad thing, as long as they are given a joyful life. The book makes us wonder what divides the human and the other-than-human. Maren Linett's approach is a posthumanist one. It appreciates the arbitrariness of species boundaries (Linett, 2020).

As 'life ethicists', we can be involved in different scientific endeavours that deal with life in general and specific life forms. Rather than accepting concepts of difference and disease from medical science as accurate, bioethicists could question these and advocate for incorporating diverse ways of being and thinking. This approach is far removed from sterile discussions about whether we can decide whose lives are worthwhile and whose are not from an external vantage point. Fiction in all its forms can help here. That does not mean that all stories are an adequate means to accomplish this. Fiction is not immune to stereotypical representations. For example, Katta Spiel and Kathrin Gerling, researchers in Human-Computer Interaction, reviewed 66 publications in HCI research on games and different forms of neurodivergence (such as autism, ADHD, dyslexia, dyspraxia) (Spiel and Gerling, 2020). They found that these publications often dealt with neurodivergence from a strictly medical model: neurodivergent players and their disabilities were often described using negative terms and concerning problems and deficits. Moreover, games aimed at a neurodiverse audience often had a hidden therapeutic aim: they were geared at teaching players specific skills under the guise of a game. Spiel and Gerling rightly state that

> the overbearing tendency towards drawing on medical arguments (without following them through methodologically or epistemologically) harms neurodivergent populations' play experience. (Spiel, 2020)

Indeed, it seems unjust that enjoyment is always a means to a (hidden) therapeutic or pedagogical end for a specific population. Maybe bioethicists also have a task to fulfil regarding the representation of the characters in the stories themselves.

Bioethics operates at the intersection of medicine, science, and humanities. We can say that there is no such thing as a bioethicist. Anyone at this intersection and taking up the role of knitting together experiences, intuitions, approaches, and theories is a bioethicist. We would do well to engage in storytelling actively. Such engagement means being inspired by fiction in the broadest sense of the world. Reading, watching, playing or listening to good fiction can show us the way towards a future worth fighting for, even when there is much trouble.

Furthermore, maybe bad fiction can teach us how not to think. Equipped with stories, the bioethicist can help scientists and clinical practitioners to think up their own stories about the technology or practice they are considering. They can engage in a creative exercise to conjure up the possible consequences of design decisions and find out whether they have a ready answer to *cui bono*.

PART FIVE
BIOETHICS

In which I suggest how to practice what I have preached

Don't let me die in an automobile

I wanna lie in an open field

Want the snakes to suck my skin

Want the worms to be my friends

Want the birds to eat my eyes

As here I lie

The Clouds Fly By

– Jim Morrison

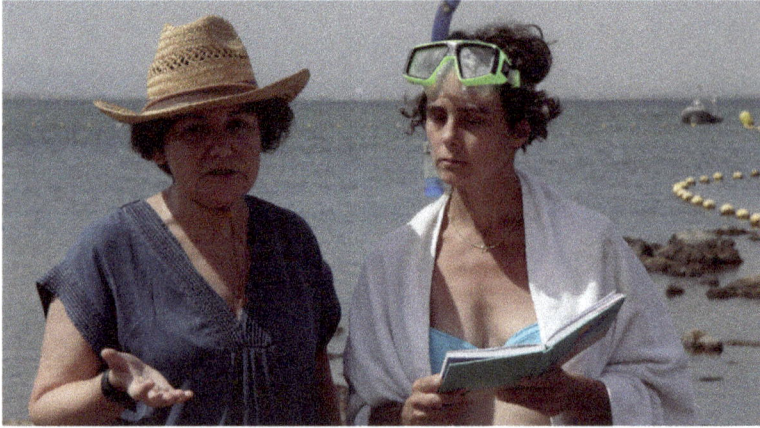

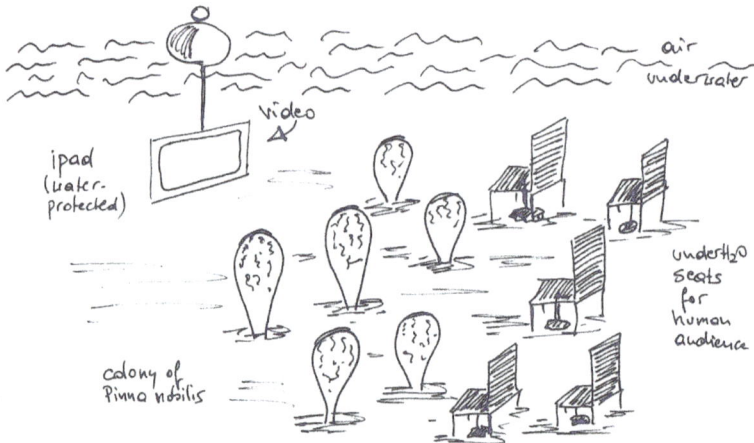

Underwater Performance for Molluscs.

Is caring for molluscs expressed by signalling them to relocate?

From: Training Program for Assisted Migration — Episode 2 *Pinna Nobilis*.
Video tutorial for molluscs; underwater performance in the Mar Menor, Spain, 2019.

Photo by Julio Daniel Suarez, 2019

Sketch by Christina Stadlbauer, 2019[1]

---

1   The Institute for Relocation of Biodiversity, Video Tutorials for Assisted Migration,
     ongoing since 2017. The complement shows an image of the performance with
     Cristina Navarro Poulin and Christina Stadlbauer introducing the human spectators
     to the idea of relocating molluscs with the help of a video tutorial. The Institute for
     Relocation of Biodiversity, Video Tutorials for Assisted Migration, ongoing since
     2017. The complement shows an image of the performance with Cristina Navarro.

So far, I have tried to summarise and link together many ideas to form a framework for forward-looking but backwards-informed bioethics. Such bioethics can help us live on a damaged planet, specifically, live well on a damaged planet. The following pages provide four other cases to illustrate this. In this concluding part, I suggest how the ideas I have described can guide the bioethicist in everyday work. These ideas relate to the necessity of engaging different standpoints (standpoint epistemology), an appreciation of the context-sensitivity of specific challenges, and the need to engage with uncertainties regarding scientific and clinical knowledge actively. One example will reflect on my work as an ethicist in a research consortium on the early detection of autism. I describe the ethical questions raised by the early detection of autism and within that specific research study. I demonstrate how a fruitful engagement with these ethical questions necessitates an engagement with ontological and epistemological questions surrounding autism. I shall describe the paradox of perhaps the most troubling ethical question: our relationship with other-than-human beings. Finally, I shall use my experiences playing a video game to tell how being open to the indeterminacy and open-endedness of ethical questions necessarily entails an active engagement with the possibility of failure and getting it wrong. Even in a (post)pandemic world where 'getting it wrong' may have catastrophic consequences, I argue that aspects of luck, uncertainty, or indeterminacy are challenging ethical reflection and opportunities that allow constant revision and reflection of conclusions.

Poulin and Christina Stadlbauer introducing the human spectators to the idea of relocating molluscs with the help of a video tutorial.

17. Concepts

Risks

Risks, and weighing them against benefits, are recurrent themes in bioethics. A medical procedure, research protocol or environmental technology that is too risky is unethical. Consider discussions surrounding the precautionary principle or 'acceptable risk' in research. Adding risk and security to the debate also elevates the discussion above the mere ethical: risk and security give a scientific flavour to ethical arguments. At the same time, sociologists and philosophers have scrutinised the seeming objectivity of risks in science. Risk is an inherently normative term. In what follows, I shall demonstrate that we must constantly question the concept of risk in bioethics. How do ethics and risks relate to one another? I teach bioethics to undergraduate biology and biochemistry students. In one lesson, I present some moral theories with their strong and weak points in the same way that many bioethicists do. There is deontology, utilitarianism, and Rawls' theory of justice. There are virtue ethics and care ethics. In the next lesson, I discuss some bioethical principles and offer a defence and a critique of principlism. At this point, when talking about specific cases and applying moral theories and principles to these cases, sometimes students would proclaim themselves to be 'utilitarian'. That seems to be the moral theory closely fitting their worldview as (future) scientists. These students believe that trying to answer whether a specific potential technology should be developed or whether a medical treatment is morally justified should be decided by weighing the pros and cons without referencing fuzzy concepts such as dignity or integrity. What do these terms mean, after all? It is easy to dismiss these utterings of students as naïve, as them not understanding what ethics is. As teachers, we can give plenty of examples of what may be wrong with utilitarianism. Philippa Foot's

 https://doi.org/10.11647/OBP.0320.17

trolley problem is a good starting point to discuss different aspects of morality, although this thought experiment has not stood the test of time. Nevertheless, the consequences of decisions do matter, and there is much to say in favour of balancing risks and benefits, especially when deciding on technologies and courses of action that will influence people's lives.

Although, specifically in present-day secular bioethics, the popularity of utilitarianism is high for reasons I have described above (clean, scientific), and although risks seem to be relevant for such calculation and morality itself, *what risks are* is often not questioned. Indeed, evaluating the risks themselves appears to be delegated to a separate realm, science, which is then situated conceptually before ethical reflection. In project proposals, risks and safety issues are things the scientists themselves will solve that have no bearing on ethics. If we, the bioethicists, need risks, for example, as an ingredient for our utilitarian calculus, we sometimes suggest that such information will, in the end, become available as science progresses. Moreover, this allows us to set aside the question of the concept of risk in that particular research project. Studying the specificities of risk will be tackled by someone else. Maybe thinking about risks and the normative decisions accompanying risk assessments is another element of the bioethicist's job. But we must do so carefully without a naïve conception of what risk and benefit mean. In what follows, I want to question the bioethicist's relation to the concept of risk and risk calculation. I will be inspired by Ulrich Beck's seminal work *Risk Society* (Beck, Lash and Wynne, 1992).

Think, for example, about the discussion surrounding reproductive decision-making. Remember the case of He Jiankui, the Chinese researcher who used embryo editing to make babies resistant to HIV. This experiment has been widely condemned for several reasons. The technology is not yet ready to allow this technology to be used safely in embryos. After all, there is a risk that the technology will also alter other parts of the DNA, leading to worse outcomes for the embryos. Maybe the technology introduced some epigenetic changes in the embryonic cells, and the effects of these changes may only be visible once the resulting babies have been born or during their lifetime. These considerations are constituents of ethical reflection.

Nevertheless, some ethicists argue that we should be prepared for these risks to be resolved by technological progress. Unquestionably we can imagine the implications of a risk-free embryo editing technique. This would provide possibilities to eradicate genetic diseases from the germline. In fact, it would probably generate other options: we could make future children resistant to certain conditions, such as HIV, or, who knows, not to be affected by contagious viruses such as COVID-19. If the procedure can be completely risk-free, we may even ensure that babies have a good start in life by giving them a better memory or intelligence. By removing any reference to risks, we invite the potential of a future where technologies that may forever be too risky are possible. By positioning it as possible, it becomes the topic of investigation for ethicists. Is it desirable to have such a disease-free future where we can decide what kind of child we want? I understand the attractiveness of this kind of reasoning. Risks, as I would argue, are messy and uncontrollable. By delegating them to the scientists for answers, we free up space to investigate the potential impact of such a 'utopian' future. We may also encounter some new and detestable dilemmas. Undoubtedly, many would say it is better to live disease-free. Provided such technology can be deployed risk-free, what reasons do we have not to use it?

Maybe there is even a duty or a 'strong argument for' prospective parents to pursue these technologies, as Oxford bioethicist Julian Savulescu would argue. A particular strength of these 'what if' scenarios is that they also allow us to question how easily such utopias present themselves as places of happiness. In utopias, well-being is primarily related to what is in our genes and embodiment. Of course, this is simplistic: what if boys or heterosexual or cisgender people have a better chance of happiness in life than those who do not fit in that description? Surely if we assume that intelligence or memory can be designed, we could CRISPR these characteristics as well? This assumption would go a bridge too far for many of my colleagues. We are confronted here with one of the significant challenges bioethics faces. Taking a simplistic, atomistic, and individualistic approach to well-being, illness, and happiness just does not cut it in the long run. It is not merely a question of the desirability of the technology alone: ethical questions are never entirely separated from questions of justice and what makes a just society. I admit that using these fictional scenarios offers one way of tackling broader issues concerning what people with all kinds of (unaltered) biologies can expect from society. Still, distilling the 'true' ethical questions from the ones related to risks and safety will not take us very far if we want to answer the question of whether certain reproductive technologies should be pursued or not. That is because deciding what counts as risk is a normative question.

Authors often distinguish between objective and subjective risks in philosophical writings on risks. Objective risks are those we can calculate and put into a risk model. In line with the CRISPR discussion, this would mean calculating the probability that a particular procedure would yield undesirable results. For example, it implies that we can calculate whether the technique would introduce new mutations in parts of the DNA that were not targeted.

Subjective risks are those we cannot calculate because they are part of the value system of individuals. However, the world of risks is more complicated than this dichotomy between subjective and objective risk would suggest. An eye-opening work is Ulrich Beck's *Risk Society* (*Risikogesellschaft*) (Beck, Lash and Wynne, 1992). Beck wrote the first edition of this book in 1986, a few months after the Chernobyl disaster. I read it in 2020 when the COVID-19 pandemic was in full force and was struck by the relevance this book still has. In *Risk Society*, Beck challenges the idea that the global risks that we encounter in modern times, such as those related to pollution and global warming, can be easily pinned down, calculated and neutralised using scientific methods. The book demonstrates the importance of sociologists and bioethicists taking each other's work seriously to form a complete picture of the issues. Risks are, to a certain extent, incalculable. They are about hypotheticals: what might happen. Hence, utilitarian calculus is almost always a jump in the dark except in the most banal circumstances. If we choose to continue to use electricity from nuclear power plants, we may alleviate global warming, but we may also risk destroying the world. We cannot weigh these two risks against one another, at least not in a definite way. Science itself will not give ultimate answers on how to deal with risk. Scientific explanations may yield an aura of calculability, but in the end, many risks are just not calculable.

Moreover, what we choose to see as a risk is not value-free. Beck points to the idea of an 'acceptable level' when dealing with, for example, pollution. He calls this 'a phoney trick': we may think there is a scientifically sound way of defining such a level, but we need only to prove that our actions yield side effects below this acceptable level to give the impression of being safe in a scientifically proven way. However, who defines these acceptable levels and on what basis? Ethicists can question these aspects of technology and not merely take for granted that the experts will tell us what acceptable risks are. Think about the example of epigenetics and pollution I gave in this book's first part. If living in polluted areas may impact you directly, surely this needs to be part of discussions about what kind of technologies or industries we find acceptable. The knowledge that this may affect future generations can complicate the questions of acceptable levels even further. Questions about our responsibilities to future generations are normative ones, not technical ones. Maybe new insights on the molecular effects of pollution may also shed some light on alleviating them. It is a critical task for ethicists and philosophers to work closely with those who have to assess these risks and question assumptions and possible solutions. With Beck, I also believe that such an approach does not need to distrust science or assume that all risks are subjective and have no basis. Beck points out that our modernity is reflexive: we relate to risks and think about them. Acknowledging that many risks are not as objectifiable as we may assume and that there is always some uncertainty about future consequences does not make science less scientific. On the contrary, I believe fruitful engagement between philosophers and scientists will make science more scientific and philosophy more relevant in the 21st century.

I have described uncertainties about weighing risks and which conclusions to draw from these calculations. There is also uncertainty about what a risk is and what happens if we call something a risk. A risk has, by definition, the connotation of something unwanted. Objectifying it in quantitative terms does not remove that connotation. I remember a discussion we had with the researchers of a project I was involved in. This project investigated the possibility of early detection of autism in young children born prematurely, who had experienced eating problems as a baby, or had a sibling diagnosed with autism. These children are considered at a higher 'risk' for autism. Hence, the project name was TIARA, a nice-sounding name with possibilities for fancy house styles. TIARA is an acronym for Tracking Infants at Risk for Autism. I was involved as the primary investigator of the ethics work package. In the project's first months, it became clear that the term 'risk' was somewhat problematic. Autistic people do not want to see themselves as a hazard. Moreover, there is an uncomfortable association between early detection and early intervention. Indeed, if something is considered a risk, projects aiming to detect these risks will aid in the prevention or at least alleviate risks. The term 'at risk for autism' seems to imply that it is the autism itself that needs to be prevented or alleviated. However, many autistic people would argue that their autism is an intrinsic part of their identity. Some would say that what needs fixing is our society and its attitudes towards those with a different neurotype. Hence, such projects should first aim to understand and enable the necessary support and understanding for the autistic way of being. We can also ask ourselves what is meant by 'being at risk for autism'. Does this mean being at risk of exhibiting the behavioural phenomena that are the prerequisites for a diagnosis? Does it mean being at risk for having a certain atypical way of information processing or sensory processing? Does it mean being at risk of suffering from these phenomena? What struck me at a given moment when discussing the problematic aspects of risk language concerning autism was that one of the researchers, a professor in psychology, stated that for them, 'risk' was a neutral term. In the sense that they used the term risk in their research, it was more or less synonymous with 'chance', the possibility that something might happen. A risk is something you calculate, and it becomes stripped of any negative connotations. It merely is. Most people, including scientists, would not go that far and would still consider risk as something that is regarded as harmful, that we want to avoid, even if we hope to control it by calculating it. Nevertheless, if we consider risk as something objective, we may assume that risk is beyond discussion. Perhaps it is the other way around: calling something a risk is creating something as a risk. It is a normative move with specific consequences, positive or negative. It is precisely this move that we should reflect upon and not take for granted. I will illustrate with some examples. My examples align with Justin Biddle and Quill Kukla's phronetic risks (Biddle and Kukla, 2017). These are defined as epistemic risks that arise during the course of activities that are preconditions for or parts of empirical (inductive or abductive) reasoning, insofar as these are risks that need to be managed and balanced in light of values and interests. (2017, p. 220)

They give the example of how scientists operationalise disease concepts and set criteria for inclusion in a disease category that will become the topic of empirical investigation. For example, if we consider the example of long COVID-19: If this phenomenon is deemed to represent a specific disease, there is an opening for it to end up in risk calculations during pandemics.

Perhaps calling something a risk is a phronetic risk: it will make certain practices inevitable and obscure further questioning about what makes the phenomena a risk. One example is risk calculations for trisomy-21. It is known that the older a woman is when she conceives, the higher the chance of the baby having trisomy-21 — Down syndrome — becomes. These higher chances are often expressed through 'risk'. It is also known that specific genetic mutations detected during pregnancy yield a higher chance of a child with a cognitive disability. Such chances are also expressed in risk factors. Based on these risk factors, clinicians decide whether to communicate this risk to prospective parents or not. Let us assume the fictitious example of a specific genetic mutation associated with cognitive disability in 1% of the cases. Many geneticists and ethicists alike would argue that this is not meaningful information and would hesitate to communicate this to pregnant women. However, just as in the case of 'a higher risk for autism', merely associating 'risk' with the resulting phenotype may obscure specific considerations that may be of personal and ethical relevance. For example, a 45-year-old woman has a 1/30 chance of having a baby with Down syndrome. Often this is written as a risk of 1/30. Let us take a closer look at what this might mean. Of course, part of the meaning of risk is related to the statistical probability: there is a 1/30 probability that this woman's child would have Down syndrome. 'Risk', however, has another more normative connotation. It may imply that a child with Down syndrome is de facto and objectively undesirable. However, this cannot be true, as prospective parents often continue with pregnancies if the child has trisomy-21. Sometimes, prospective parents choose not to undergo prenatal testing because 'any child is welcome'. Moreover, besides the ethical connotations, regarding

Trisomy-21 as a 'risk' seems ontologically problematic, as indeed the condition is equated with 'a person with Down syndrome'. It is not an accidental characteristic of a person. We cannot think of trisomy-21 as separate from a specific person with Down syndrome. Indeed, it is odd to view persons with specific identity-defining characteristics as risks and even more peculiar to say that the risk is that a particular type of people will be born.

Perhaps 'a risk for Down syndrome' means something else. Metonymically, it may look like it refers to the person in question, but we are actually referring to the undesirable effects associated with Down syndrome. It is here that unreflective risk talk becomes ethically problematic. By shortcutting all conceivable risks associated with Down syndrome into one package—'the risk for Down syndrome'—the specific particularities that we think are risks remain hidden for ethical scrutiny. At this point in the debate, I can imagine clinicians starting to refer to the increased chance of people with Down syndrome having certain heart conditions. It makes sense to say that people with Down syndrome have a 30% more risk of having certain heart conditions that require intervention and surgery when they are babies. I think the use of risk is wholly warranted here. But the risk of 'having a child with Down syndrome' and the risk of 'that a baby with Down syndrome needs surgery' are not at the same level. We cannot readily say that they mean the same thing. We need to dissect better what is meant by the first utterance. The oft-stated association with health problems such as heart conditions and shorter life span already shows us the way to such dissection. It becomes clear that the implied risk means several things. First, the most obvious one is that people assume that the well-being of people with Down syndrome is less than that of others. What is at risk here is that a person will be born with a suboptimal quality of life. This is an understandable worry but one that is empirically testable. Several empirical studies suggest that the well-being of people with Down syndrome, or their parents or siblings for that matter, is comparable to that of people without Down syndrome. We can safely assume that what we are risking cannot be synonymous with the risk of giving birth to a person with a diminished chance of a happy life, although intuitively, people might think that is the case. Another risk that is often quoted is related to societal support.

Prospective parents may argue that they understand that, in principle, a child with Down syndrome has a chance for a happy life just like anybody else. Still, they may be afraid that the child will be severely bullied. Alternatively, they may worry about what will happen if they die and the child outlives them. Will they wither away in state institutions? Will the burden of care fall on any surviving siblings who were never included in the decision-making process in the first place? It is often these worries about the future that people think about when they imagine giving birth to a child with Down syndrome. However, such considerations are categorically different from considerations related to the child's well-being. It is safe to say that children with Down syndrome are not, by definition, unhappier or have less well-being than children without Down syndrome. Some may be happier, and others may be unhappier, just like everyone has individual differences. Ethical considerations based on assumptions regarding the well-being and happiness of those who have not been born yet are often misguided, and ethicists should avoid them. But considerations that have to do with the lack of support for people with disabilities and their parents are fundamentally different. Considering these should not automatically lead to the conclusion that Down syndrome is a risk that should be avoided. True, at a given time or place where support for people with Down syndrome or societal acceptance is terrible, this may be a good reason prospective parents would choose not to give birth to such a child. Hence, the societal nature of the 'risk' per se is not a straightforward reason why the conclusion should be that parents do not have the right to make these choices. For ethicists, such conceptual dissection of what risk means can be an eye-opener that these considerations should not be solely based on individual risks but are related to the broader society. It reveals that these choices are embedded in contexts that in themselves are unjust. At the same time, it calls for a reassessment of how we look at disability.

At least two other meanings can be implied in 'a risk for Down syndrome'. Prospective parents may fear the burden that raising such a child may put on their families. They may worry that they are not up to raising a disabled child, although they know that Down syndrome children can also have rich and fulfilling lives. They may think they are not the right people to provide this life for them. These worries could also be connected to society's lack of support for families with disabled children. It may be related to unreasonable fears about this support. Such concerns demonstrate that prospective parents should be given accurate information about available support and what life is like with a disabled child to alleviate this fear. It may very well be the case that these fears are founded and that the societal circumstances are such that parents of disabled children are unreasonably burdened. For example, it may be unavoidable that at least one parent will have to give up their professional hopes and dreams, which in turn may bring financial pressure, which may be an even more significant consideration than losing a career. Reproductive ethics should not solely consider which individual choices we can make available. There is a need for reflection on the broader societal context. Rather than condemning or applauding parents' decision-making, bioethicists can also actively advocate for just and inclusive societies. Such a society is one where people can welcome disabled children into their families without worrying about giving up their careers or ending up in financial hardships. Some would consider this a political or ideological stance. I guess this is unavoidable.

Nevertheless, and now we are moving into more contentious arguments, the risk for Down syndrome that prospective parents consider may not be related to support or happiness. It may be the case that some parents have a very perfectionist dream about what their children should be like. The risk they face when thinking about future offspring is that the child they will have will not live up to their dreams. The likelihood that a child with Down syndrome will attend an Ivy League university could be lower than for a child without Down syndrome. Some people may attach so much importance to specific characteristics of their future children that a child with a disability just does not fit this vision. The majority of the literature does not deal with such difficult questions. Arguments like these are often disguised by references to the well-being of the children themselves. When scholars discuss reproductive technologies to prevent Down syndrome, they usually refrain from the thought that some people would prefer to have children with a higher likelihood of fulfilling specific dreams. The often-vague reference to risks suggests that avoiding a child with a disability is self-evident. It is assumed that this is better for everyone, including the never-to-be-born potential children themselves. In a certain way, this is understandable. Very few prospective parents or clinicians will have one specific and well-articulated reason why they think it is best not to proceed with certain pregnancies. Motivations and feelings are messy: people can simultaneously believe that the child will become unhappy, be bullied, and feel that this is not the future they had imagined they would have with their families. We cannot expect prospective parents to perform an ethical analysis of all their arguments and check them against empirical truths to come to one transparent and ethical decision. It is the task of biomedical ethicists to make sure that ethical analysis about such matters is clear-cut. Ethicists can shed light on the different levels of analysis and complexities at stake. Still, some ethicists feel that there is something morally wrong if prospective parents choose not to have a specific child because the child would not conform to their respective aesthetic or intellectual ideals. Authors have used a virtue ethics approach to condemn such practices in this respect. They would argue that accepting children as they are is what makes someone a good parent. I am sympathetic to this view. However, I also think this is not an argument we can readily use to discuss prenatal diagnosis. There are several reasons for that. First, we may think that such parents (or those who may want to engineer embryos to have beautiful children, for that matter) somehow fail in one respect of what makes one a good parent. However, this does not mean that they are overall bad parents. What makes someone a good parent is hard to define. It changes over time and cannot be pinned to one characteristic alone. The same people could be excellent parents for their dream child, for all we know. Second, as I have already hinted, the reasoning and arguments behind prenatal choices are seldomly clear-cut. Overall, they will be a mixture of well-being considerations, the perceived care and financial burden to the family and the loss of hopes and dreams regarding one's future children. Thirdly, even if the decision to end a pregnancy is because of cosmetic concerns or because people believe their child should have strong cognitive skills, it is difficult to use the ideal of the virtuous parent to forbid it. Should we argue in favour of an unborn, unwanted child and say that it is better to be born unwanted than not born at all? This implies arguing that denying the termination of a pregnancy is more important than the right to a woman's reproductive autonomy. In any case, assessing the motivations behind reproductive decisions is problematic precisely because of their messiness. However, that does not mean we, as bioethicists, must think such choices are morally unproblematic. It is essential to acknowledge that what we advocate for, such as reproductive autonomy, can be ethically problematic in other aspects and can go against our moral intuitions or conscience. At the same time, this is insufficient ground to forbid or argue against something.

Another type of risk is associated with the statement 'risk for Down syndrome'. It is a risk that is sensitive and tricky to acknowledge. However, if we want a clear view of the task of the bioethicist, we need to face it. People may mean that there is a risk for Down syndrome because there is a risk that a child will be born who will burden society. Few would openly admit that this is the reason for the widespread availability of prenatal screening programmes. In most cases, such screening programmes are presented as having a primary aim of enhancing prospective parents' reproductive autonomy. Prenatal diagnosis is offered to people to decide for themselves whether they are up to raising a child with a specific disability. However, the cost of disabled persons to society may have played a role when such programmes were first discussed. It is possible to find papers in the health economy that compare the rollout of a non-invasive prenatal screening programme for Down syndrome with the lifetime cost of supporting people with Down syndrome (Ohno and Caughey, 2013).

Nevertheless, on the whole, policymakers and reproductive specialists alike would consider it an unsavoury idea that the rollout of prenatal screening programmes is primarily a cost-saving operation.[2]

---

2   I have encountered this argument at least twice. One was in an interview study with couples undergoing fertility treatement for chromosomal translocations. These chromosomal abnormalities lowered the chance of conceiving naturally. Sometimes, these translocations could also lead to the birth of a child with disabilities. When discussing the selection of embryos with disabilities, some of my respondents stated that they thought they shouldn't bring a disabled child into this world, precisely because they had already used public health funding to become pregnant. They felt that because of that, it would be unethical to bring a child into this world that would burden the public health system even more (Hens *et al.*, 2019). Another time was when my university had invited the British bioethicist John Harris for a lecture. John Harris and I agreed to disagree about disability rights, and the lecture was mainly about internet security and privacy. But as John Harris is also known for his stance on reproductive ethics (see for example Harris, 2005), and has argued in some papers that it is better not to bring disabled people into this world, the audience had questions about this as well. It struck me that several people from the audience thought that the idea that we must not bring disabled people into

Still, we must tackle this possible interpretation of what it means to 'risk' a Down syndrome child. This is the 'risk' that a child is born that will be a burden to the health care system. The question here is whether we should accept this as a possible interpretation of 'risk for Down syndrome'. I argue that it is not. I admit it may be hard to find arguments for this. The questions of what kind of society we want and what we can expect from members of this society are political and possibly ideological ones. It may be possible to argue that a society that takes care of and invests in its most vulnerable members is a better society than one that wants to eliminate all kinds of vulnerabilities. Opponents could argue that it is precisely because we eliminate as many vulnerabilities as possible before they arise, for example, by ensuring that vulnerable children are not born, we safeguard funding for those who become vulnerable later. As a counterargument, we can suggest that a diverse society is better than one with only people who conform to a certain standard of health or autonomy. The argument of preventing Down syndrome children because they would cost too much to society is unacceptable to me. At the same time, I believe we must respect the individual choices of parents, and their considerations regarding their own finances or the well-being of existing children can be valid.

The bioethicist's task may be to provide narratives to the public which illuminate the rich lives disabled people live without judging individual choices and safeguarding women's right to bodily integrity. They may help demonstrate that framing disability, especially cognitive disability, primarily a burden for society is misguided. A stubborn refusal to acknowledge these lived experiences and alternative narratives, as some have done, is exhibiting bad faith. Analysing what we mean when we say 'a risk for Down syndrome' does not straightforwardly lead to an ethical answer as to whether it is right to terminate a pregnancy if the foetus has trisomy-21. I believe it is not the bioethicist's task to provide such an answer. Instead, their task is to make sure that clinicians and policymakers alike are aware of these possible interpretations, the

---

this world because they cost too much money for the health care system (which is, as far as I understand it, not Harris's approach) is a perfectly valid argument. I think we cannot blame these prospective parents for thinking that way (unlike the bioethicists, who I think we can actually blame), but it is a sign of what people feel they 'owe' to society that has helped them in certain ways.

appeals for justice and the possible misinterpretations of disability they lay bare. As such, they can enable more informed choices.

At the time of writing this chapter, the COVID-19 pandemic is in full force. In Belgium, where I live, we are on the verge of a third wave. In this pandemic, the uncertainty of what counts as a risk and which risks we should include in calculations that form the basis of policies is ongoing. Because the question of risk in a pandemic is complex, there is a tendency to reduce risk calculation to a mere technocratic approach. What we risk is then defined as risk for transmission or mortality risk. Nevertheless, the pandemic has made it abundantly clear that it is impossible to make a policy for lockdowns or other measures based on these technical risks alone. On the one hand, with a lockdown, we risk incurring other risks: loss of income for those dependent on patronages, such as hotels, pubs, hairdressers and restaurants (Schaubroeck and Hens, 2021). If schools are closed, we may drastically reduce transmission rates, but children miss out on education, which in itself is correlated with a lower life expectancy, so it seems (Hummer and Hernandez, 2013). On the other hand, the risks of the disease itself are not well known and may depend on the specific individual and their context. Some people risk having long-term consequences, and it is not entirely clear who incurs the highest risk for these.

The loss of smell and taste for months on end that many people experience may be a small price to pay for freedom and may not warrant the lockdown. At the same time, such loss is devastating if you are a sommelier or a chef. Ulrich Beck's analysis of the risk society and global risks seems more relevant than ever: a mere technological approach to risk will not automatically lead to just policies, and tackling one 'risk' may beget others (Beck, Lash and Wynne, 1992). It would be naive to think that bioethicists can solve ethical dilemmas in pandemics. But we can keep pointing out the different aspects of risks and how various risks cannot be reduced or even weighed against one another. We operate in a mode of uncertainty, and acknowledging or uncovering that fact may be helpful.

18. Development

Autism Research

In the first part of this book, I spent much time explaining how a developmental view of life can complement or even replace more mechanistic approaches that are gene-centric and perhaps even reductionist. Such a developmental view is not new. It goes back to age-old discussions about how organisms get their forms. Over the last decades, present-day findings regarding genetics and epigenetics and the gut microbiome's role in health and personality have given us a far more nuanced view of organisms. Such a view complements and extends what is available in the classic 'modern synthesis' of the twentieth century, which may have taken the life out of biology. We are gaining back a view of biology teeming with life, small and big. Besides selfish genes, which still play an—albeit minor—role, this view on biology is full of cooperating entities, chance encounters and unexpected opportunities. By definition, and in the words of Stuart Kauffman, life is unprestatable. To understand it, we must relinquish the idea that we can ultimately control it. What we get, in return, is a future where many opportunities are still open. A future that we can also, to some extent, create ourselves. Still, we cannot deny that 'biology' has different connotations and works in specific ways to evaluate certain phenomena. Biology makes something real, which gives credibility to one's experiences. I am reminded here of an interview study I did with adults who had received a recent diagnosis of autism (Hens and Langenberg, 2018). According to my research participants, the fact that autism was so firmly linked to something neurological and genetic was helpful. It made their experiences authentic and credible. If we insist on a more dynamic, processual view of life, are we not losing precisely that? I have

 https://doi.org/10.11647/OBP.0320.18

suggested elsewhere that bringing back a more dynamic perspective on biology can help thinking about neurodevelopmental phenomena—such as autism—differently: it can reposition the developmental condition of autism as something genuinely developmental. In what follows, I will reflect on what such an approach may mean for autism research.

Autism is conceived in scientific literature and by autistic people as tightly linked with genes and biology. Genes are often conceptualised as information about a certain, or at least probable, future. We do not yet know everything there is to know about genes, but if science progresses, we will. In bioethics, this line of thinking is sometimes taken for granted. Discussions are often of the format 'what if we can select an embryo for intelligence' or 'should we test for autism genes prenatally', usually implying that the discussion is really whether autism is a good reason for a termination of pregnancy. Nevertheless, recent findings in epigenetics and microbiomics, together with the fact that genetic knowledge has not delivered on its promise, suggest that this idea of genetic predictions and determination is naive. Biology is not fixed. It is dynamic, in the same way our personalities and identities are defined by the relationships we form. Throughout our lives, we are thoroughly influenced, and we influence what and who we encounter. We are entangled with our physical and biological environment. The new science of epigenetics, gene expression, is reminiscent of epigenesis, which refers to development. Furthermore, development is not just what happens in the first three years of our lives: it occurs from birth until we die. Bioethicists must not solely slavishly follow where biomedical science leads them but question the assumption of science itself. We can also play a role in advocating for a developmental approach to autism research. For decades, researchers have sought to explain autism through genetic analysis. That is understandable: biological explanations can give insight into one's functioning, strength, and challenges. Nobody denies that biology has a role in understanding phenomena such as autism. For decades, this explanation has been sought in the genes. This genetic crusade was a reaction to earlier psychogenic explanations that were stigmatising for parents. For example, in the fifties, psychoanalysts' explanations for autism would refer to the cold behaviour of mothers toward their child as the origin of autism. As a result, many autistic children were institutionalised, and their parents were left feeling blamed and stigmatized. Today, early detection research often consists of finding a gene or another biomarker that can detect and predict autism presymptomatically. Moreover, a genetic explanation has the advantage that the idea that 'it is in your genes' is linked with your identity, with who you are, rather than with what you have experienced or what your parents might have done to you.

There certainly is value in genetic research to understand biological mechanisms better. Nevertheless, with the search for genetic explanations, we miss an opportunity to understand autistic people and their interaction with the physical, biological and social environment. The opposition between static biology and dynamic experience is a false one. We discussed that at length when we talked about developmental systems theory and the ideas of Georges Canguilhem. In early detection research, which aims to predict the possibility of an autism diagnosis later in life, it is sometimes unclear what the aims are. Initially, it was often sold as alleviating or curing autism, a purpose we would not accept any more. Conversely, early detection research may have the noble aim of accommodating differences proactively. However, detection based on biomarkers alone only yields an understanding outside of context and situations. It can only be partial. Strikingly, autism belongs to the category of developmental conditions, implying that certain atypicalities happen during a specific developmental window early in life. Atypicalities that, if detected early enough, we could alleviate or even set straight. However, studying autism as a developmental phenomenon in a different, a more epigenetic sense may be more fruitful or even more ethical. It is a fact that autism has different and dynamic meanings for the individual throughout a lifetime. Truly understanding autism and autistic people means being ready to study them and their experiences throughout their lifetime, listening to their stories, and their sense-making in a specific relational context. Moreover, a dynamic approach to life is not only bidirectional. It means that research goals can be adaptive. This is especially true for clinical research that, we may hope, ultimately aims to make people's lives better. Ethical autism research is thus research that is co-created with autistic people and their families from its inception.

I have argued that a genuinely scientific science of autism is not only about ultimate causes. However, to study autistic people and their experiences over a lifetime, there need to be structural changes in how science and research projects are funded. A typical research project is four years long. This is just enough to fund a PhD student to do the work. Understandably, people focus on quick wins, such as the statistical association of a specific gene with a particular phenotype; or a molecular finding in a family with a specific phenotype that includes an autism diagnosis. At the same time, science has an ethical imperative to seek the best and most complete understanding of the world. Alongside this fragmented knowledge that genes can yield, science must also zoom out and look at interactions and developments. Furthermore, as we have seen, philosophers of science such as Ian Hacking, Bruno Latour and new materialist scholars such as Karen Barad show us that science is not only a representation of external reality. It also creates realities. This insight implies an ethical appeal in 'doing' science: do it right and make the right choices. If we look at autism research in the past, much has gone wrong. Theories that have tried to explain autism, such as the theory that autistic people would have a deficit in Theory of Mind, or assumptions that autistic people would lack empathy, have created a context that was actively harmful to autistic people. They were set apart as not belonging to 'us', the typically functioning people. Ethicists and philosophers of science must not take scientific practice for granted but query its conceptual assumptions and the realities it creates. From a genuinely developmental and ethical perspective, a science looking at autism, or any other phenomena, must value individual experiences and differences above generalisations about autistic people and their functioning or assumptions about how their minds might work. Methods traditionally used in biomedical research, such as statistical methods and comparison of biomarker measurements, are not sufficient. The experiences of autistic people are pivotal to understanding autism. Hence, an actual science of autism is interdisciplinary, valuing input from the humanities and other sciences. It means engaging with autistic people, employing autistic researchers, and actively collaborating on methods to incorporate experiences from those traditionally left out of specific research, such as people with non-standard communication preferences. To do so, arts-based methods, such as the one Leni Van Goidsenhoven used when thinking with a young woman who communicated in non-traditional ways, can be an important part of research endeavours across disciplines (Van Goidsenhoven and De Schauwer, 2020). Artistic methods can help open up new possibilities for understanding life in all its diversity, and art and science can complement each other and develop new opportunities for knowledge. Cooperation with the humanities is integral to a holistic science that tries to understand phenomena in all their nuances and dynamics. Furthermore, insisting on this approach in specific research projects is not enough. Ethicists have a vital role in advocating for a reform of research funding and publication practices that makes research more ready for the challenges we will be facing in the upcoming decades. Paradoxically, this means more room should be made for non-traditional, longitudinal research that tries to understand phenomena in their temporality, not just quick fixes or quick explanations.

19. Trouble

Crocodiles and Mice

A topic integral to every self-respecting bioethics course is the human relationship with other-than-human animals. We usually discuss utilitarian approaches ('do they suffer?'), deontological approaches ('are other-than-human animals subjects of a life or not? What characteristics do they need to have to be considered so?') and perhaps even care ethics approaches, for example, when teaching ethics to veterinarians. However, an ethics of care does not provide straightforward answers about what should be good care. When it comes to what we owe to animals, a care ethic approach may give the impression that it only applies to those we have in our care. This conflicts with the view that animals should not be in our care, we are not their shepherds, and they are not our property. Ethical questions regarding the rights of animals are prime examples of how bioethics should stay with the trouble of unsolvable conflicts and duties. Staying with the trouble is not defeatist. It tackles difficult questions and tragedies head-on and acknowledges that paradoxes are part of ethics. We cannot explain away the paradoxes but reflecting on them may show us the way to a more liveable future for other-than-human animals.

Bioethics is often associated with autonomy, beneficence, non-maleficence, justice, solidarity, integrity, and dignity. These principles are interpreted either as being universal or as being culturally relative. We get into trouble when we try to widen the scope of our moral considerations beyond what is human. Many of us would agree that a principle such as non-maleficence applies to how we treat animals. For many of us, including myself, this entails abstaining from eating meat. At the same time, we are confronted with predation in the wild. How do

     https://doi.org/10.11647/OBP.0320.19

we come to terms with the fact that other-than-human animals need to eat others? Some ethicists have concluded that humans should intervene to ensure that predation in the wild does not occur anymore. At the same time, there is also a body of knowledge about plant cognition and fungi cognition. What does a plant know?, as the eponymous book by David Chamovitz asks (Chamovitz, 2012). Quite a lot, it seems. If plants are aware of one another, does this mean that we should also assign them rights? Meat eaters have often confronted vegetarians for their inconsistency: surely, if it matters to you what an oyster or a mussel feels, you must consider what plants experience. How can we stay with the trouble and acknowledge that there is predation in nature, that there may be other forms of cognition than animal cognition, and still be able to advocate for the abolition of meat-eating by human beings? If we desire our ethics to be consistent and foolproof, this is the paradox we should dissolve.

An illuminating work that engages with the question of predation and our relation with nature is Val Plumwood's *The Eye of the Crocodile* (Plumwood, 2012). In this short work, freely available online, Plumwood talks about her experience of almost being eaten by a crocodile in Australia's Kakadu National Park in February 1985. This experience led to the insight that we as humans are meat. She writes:

> It is not a minor or inessential feature of our human existence that we are food: juicy, nourishing bodies. Yet, as I looked into the eye of the crocodile, I realised that my planning for this journey upriver had given insufficient attention to this important aspect of human life, to my own vulnerability as an edible, animal being. (p. 11)

As Plumwood experiences first-hand, we are food in the crocodile's eye. As such, we are an intricate part of the ecosystem surrounding us. Plumwood suggests that we should accept that fact: 'both I and the culture that shaped my consciousness were wrong, profoundly wrong—about many things, but especially about human embodiment, animality and the meaning of human life' (p. 12). Human beings have sought to deny that we are bodies made of flesh in different ways. The Cartesian split between soul and body may be a prime example: our selves—our souls—are apart from our bodies: they are eternal. As many scholars envisaged, the afterlife suggests that the decaying bodies we leave behind are nothing more than shells. People sometimes prefer to be cremated because they cannot stand the idea of being food for worms. Nevertheless, Plumwood says, Descartes was wrong: we live in a Heraclitean universe. We are part of the flow of things, not above them: just like plants, fungi and other-than-human animals, we participate in the ever-continuing flow of eating and being eaten. That is a good thing, as acknowledging that opens up possibilities for a new ecological awareness:

> The eye of the crocodile also provides us with a perspective that can help us to see ourselves in ecological terms; help us towards a theory of ourselves in thoroughgoing evolutionary–democratic terms, disrupting our view of ourselves as set apart and special. We need to respond rationally to the environmental crisis by adopting a much more ecologically democratic position. From such a viewpoint we can love fellow humans without needing to maintain an exclusionary stance towards non-humans. (Plumwood, 2012, p. 16)

In such a view, death and being eaten should not solely be seen as a tragedy or something we need to overcome. Death is a testimony that we are part of the environment that nourishes us and that, in the end, we will also nourish.

In a discussion on animal ethics, Plumwood juxtaposes this Heraclitean universe where we are part of the food chain and the universe of individual justice. The latter sees human beings as separate from their surroundings and governed by moral principles such as autonomy, beneficence, and justice. Plumwood argues that many contemporary debates on animal ethics and rights take the latter universe as a starting point. We extend principles towards the animal kingdom, or at least towards those animals with which we can identify. In this respect, animals are bearers of rights because they can experience pleasure and pain and have their own goals. Nevertheless, we live in both universes and are simultaneously prey and part of the ecological system. However, at the same time, we care about animals and want to do them justice. With Haraway, I would say we must stay with the trouble of thinking these two realities together. In this view, it makes no sense to condemn predation entirely, such as predation by subsistence hunters or wild animals. At the same time, it would also be wrong to use predation as an argument for the status quo regarding meat eating. Haraway suggests that we consider animals as kin, and the existence of predation can never be an excuse for the maltreatment of animals. Plumwood writes:

> To do so acknowledges the tension between them and acknowledges us as beings who live in both worlds. To acknowledge the soul of our food is to acknowledge that both we ourselves and what we eat belong to both worlds; it is to try to bring these worlds into harmony at the point where they touch. This is also the point where what we eat morally touches our lives. It is the point at which we have to do right by our food and acknowledge its generosity. (Plumwood, p. 39)

However, this is not the end of the argument. It would be wrong to consider the sphere of morality, care, love and justice as solely belonging to human culture and the Heraclitean universe as solely that of nature. Plumwood wants to do away with the dichotomy between nature and culture; between them and us; and with the idea that in humans alone, our bodies belong to nature, and our minds belong to culture.

> Our conviction that 'we' live in culture and 'they' live in nature is so strong that all that is left is a passionate story about consciousness, history and freedom—about us—and another story about fiercely uninvolved causation and clockwork—a story about them. (Plumwood, 2012, p. 44)

Plumwood writes how also in the natural world, there is a sense of the other as other, not merely as meat. The crocodile can view others as individuals. Morality and ethics do not only belong to human beings. Individual rules and compassion are parts of other-than-human nature as well. Recognizing this commonality is the first step toward a new kind of ethics. Concerning animal ethics, she, therefore, advocates *ecological animalism*, which

> supports and celebrates animals and encourages a dialogical ethics of sharing and negotiation or partnership between humans and animals, while undertaking a re-evaluation of human identity that affirms inclusion in animal and ecological spheres. (Plumwood, 2012, p. 78)

She juxtaposes this position against ontological veganism, which maintains the duty to abstain from all meat-eating but neglects the fact that we are also food, that we are part of a nature that is in flux, of eating and being eating. At the same time, Plumwood's approach does not justify large-scale meat-eating and the instrumentalisation of animals: by recognising ourselves as part of the food chain, we can appreciate animals and the natural world at large as kin, in a mutually dependent relationship, with reverence. Hence, many, if not all, of the current meat-eating practices are also wrong in an ecological animalism approach. Acknowledging both seemingly paradoxical aspects of human and other-than-human lives does not call for a resolution of the paradox. Neither should humanity continue indulging in industrial meat-eating because some other-than-human animals eat meat nor should we feed the lion a vegetarian diet. Paradoxes illustrate that morality is no simple zero-sum game or puzzle. It acknowledges the world's muddiness and the impossibility of keeping our boots clean. One of the most paradoxical and pressing issues that bioethicists are confronted with is the acceptability of animal experimentation.

The first chapter in John Berger's *Why Look at Animals* is about a man with mice in his house (Berger, 2009). Every morning, he notices that mice have been eating his bread. So, the protagonist sets out to buy mice traps, but they are no longer available in the local shop. He resorts to using an improvised mousetrap lying around in the house. This trap consists of a small cage, and mice are caught but not killed. When he catches his first mouse, the contraption allows him to look at the mouse in a way that he has never looked at mice. He thinks they vaguely resemble kangaroos with their strong hind legs. He looks at their behaviour in the cage and when he releases them in the field. He even gives one mouse a name, Alfredo. When the last mouse is caught, and his house is mouse-free, he realises that he will miss them. He has learned how to look at mice and see them for the wondrous beings they are, which is much more than vermin or tools for researchers to use. Mice and rats are killed by the thousands each year in animal experiments. In 2020, in Flanders, the Dutch-speaking part of Belgium, 126.797 mice were used in experiments and 9.937 rats.[1] The number of animals used in research decreases yearly and demonstrates the ethical sensitivity of using animals. However, animal experimentation is seen as regrettable yet, in some cases, unavoidable. Bioethics classes have an obligatory section about Animal Experimentation, in which we teach students about the three R's: Replacement - the substitution of conscious, living animals with insentient material where possible; Reduction—reducing

---

1   https://assets.vlaanderen.be/image/upload/v1636360925/Statistieken_proefdieren_2020_olo6oq.pdf

the number of animals used; and Refinement - any decrease in the incidence or severity of inhumane procedures applied to those animals which still must be used. W. M. S. Russell laid down these principles in R. L. Burch in 1959 (Russell and Burch, 1959)

What is not questioned in the three Rs is whether using other-than-human animals for human purposes should, in principle, be considered 'morally good'. It is perhaps easier for certain non-secular bioethicists to refer to human beings as the top of all creation, even spiced with a tinge of naturalism. For example, in a volume on personalist bioethics, Elio Sgreccia and colleagues state that the ontological and axiological difference between human beings and other living beings is one of the principles of what they call ontological bioethics. They argue, for example, that the idea of pain cannot be applied to man and animal in the same way because 'animals suffer and man [sic] knows that he suffers and seeks meaning in suffering' (Sgreccia, 2012, p. 323). For people like me, who do not have such a clear view of who suffers the most and whose suffering matters the most, such arguments do not work. For experimenters working in close contact with animals, it does not either, as is apparent from this quote by Nicholas P. Money when looking back on his life's work as a biologist.

> As a young scientist, I spent a brief spell experimenting on squid, which required me to hold the animals in my hand and feel them writhe before decapitating the poor creatures with a pair of razor-sharp surgical scissors. This was necessary to isolate the fat nerve cell called the giant axon, which is very useful for studying the transmission of nerve impulses. There was no value for a student in this foray towards vivisection. The workings of the 'action potential' can be grasped by anyone with a modicum of intelligence and access to a physiology textbook: sodium out -> depolarisation, potassium in -> repolarisation, followed by overshoot and recovery. Did my victims feel the quickening pulse in my fingers before squirting ink in a desperate bid for life? The fields of neurology and cardiology have rested for centuries on animal torture. (Money, 2021, p. 39)

Animal experiments are often presented in a kind of lifeboat situation. If we do not do animal experiments, ill children will die. However, a great many experiments are not of much practical use. As Money argues in the quote above, many of the science that animal experiments are supposed to prove do not need proof at all. Vinciane Despret gives several examples in her book *What Would Animals Say if We Asked the Right Questions?* (Despret, 2016). In chapter S for Separation, she describes unbearably cruel deprivation experiments with animal mothers and their children that set out to 'prove' that young animals suffer from being deprived of motherly care and that animal mothers will go to great lengths, even at their own detriment, to save their young. (Despret, 2016, p. 158)

I think we have it all wrong when dealing with animal experimentation. At their core, the 3 Rs we teach our students still assume that animal experimentation, because it is seemingly unavoidable, must be ethical. After all, we want medicine to progress and human children to be saved. This assumption presupposes a black-and-white view of morality and the impossibility of simultaneously holding at least two seemingly conflicting views. These views are that animal experimentation, to some extent, in the current time frame, is unavoidable, and at the same time, it is profoundly and fundamentally morally problematic. Acknowledging that using other-than-human animals for research is deeply troubling is not the same as stating that we must never sacrifice human animals. The realm of morality is not a zero-sum game. The idea is not to find the right solution to a moral puzzle. Animal experimentation is an example of where bioethicists, provided they want to be involved and stay with the trouble, must keep asking the question 'for whom does OncoMouse die', as is so succinctly stated by Donna Haraway (Haraway, 1997). As gadflies, we must keep asking the question, *cui bono*, why are we doing this? What knowledge do we get from this, and is this knowledge significant? If other-than-human animals are sacrificed, the very least we could strive for is that they die for causes that benefit humans and other-than-human beings. I will end here with a rather lengthy quote by Haraway that captures it all:

> Following Susan Leigh Star's (1991) lead, the question I want to ask my sibling species, a breast-endowed cyborg like me, is simple: Cui bono? For whom does OncoMouse TM live and die? If s/he is a figure in the strong sense, then s/he collects up the whole people. S/he is significant. That makes such a question as cui bono? Unavoidable. Who lives and dies — human, nonhuman, and cyborg-and how, because OncoMouse TM exists? What does OncoMouse TM offer when, between 1980 and 1991, death rates in the United States for African American women from breast cancer increased by 21 percent, while death rates for white women remained the same. Both groups showed a slight increase in incidence of

the disease. Who fits the standard that OncoMouse TM and her successors embody? Does s/he contribute to deeper equality, keener appreciation of heterogeneous multiplicity, and stronger accountability for liveable worlds? Is s/he a promising figure, this utterly artifactual, self-moving organism? Is the suffering caused to the research organism balanced by the relief of human suffering? What would such balance mean, and how should the question inflect practices in the machine-tool industry of science — that is, designing research protocols? These questions cannot have simple, single or final answers. (Haraway, 1997, p. 113)

Cui bono, for whom do OncoMouse and her heirs live and die. That is the question bioethicists have to ask time and again.

20. Creativity

A Game Inspiring A Bioethicist[1]

Death Stranding, a video game by Hideo Kojima, tells the story of a devastated USA and humanity on the brink of falling victim to the sixth extinction. The main character, which you control, is Sam Porter Bridges. The outside world has become dangerous, with toxic rainfall, ghouls, and terrorists. Defying danger, Sam's (and your) task is to deliver cargo to the survivors sheltering in underground buildings throughout the landscape. You create connections between people, rebuild roads, and bring joy to the preppers receiving their packages. The game was released in the autumn of 2019, but commentators have noticed the eerie resemblance to the 2020–2021 pandemic, where essential workers had to confront the infectious outside world to deliver goods to those staying inside. Admittedly, the world depicted in the game is vastly more broken than ours is right now. Nevertheless, the pandemic has made us reflect on humanity's ability to deal with catastrophe and has urged us to reconsider our fragility and responsibility in light of global collapse.

Writing a philosophical piece on *Death Stranding* seems like knocking on an open door. The game is steeped in philosophical reflection and speculation. Hideo Kojima has created a game that reflects on trauma and healing, connection, and the nature of biology. It raises questions about ectogenesis and male pregnancy, the nature of sexuality, and experiments on foetuses. The back story is filled with ponderings about the origins of life, the universe, and the links between life and death. It may be a bit too much for some, and one may wonder why an academic philosopher and bioethicist has spent 177 hours of her free time to gain all the game's trophies. In what follows, I shall explain why I thought

---

1   This is a modified version of a text that has appeared on the 'And Philosophy' blog.

    https://doi.org/10.11647/OBP.0320.20

this game was brilliant and why I believe it offers a playable example of Donna Haraway's idea of staying with the trouble, as she described it in the eponymous book. Specifically, I will focus on our relationship with technology and nature, the importance of play, failure and getting on, and the possibility of taking responsibility in the wake of catastrophe.

Possible answers to climate change's nearly unavoidable and destructive consequences can be subdivided into two big categories. First, there is the ecomodernist idea that technofixes will save us. Technology and science, so it is thought, will find a solution to present-day wicked problems if we invest enough time, money, and energy. This can either be done through geoengineering the climate or devising CO_2-neutral means of clean energy production. We may even genetically engineer ourselves, our plants, and our animals to be less resource-intensive or better able to withstand climate change's consequences. Second, there is the idea that we must return to a more pristine and natural way of living. Adherents of the latter stance believe that technology has led us towards the situation we are in now. It has led to alienation and hubris. In this view, we humans are the scourge of the earth, parasites that need to find their proper place again.

In the first view, technology is the solution, and nature is what is to be overcome. In the second view, technology is the enemy, and nature is what we should revere. Both approaches seem to be opposed to one another concerning their proposed solutions. Nevertheless, it appears that both approaches share one common assumption about the position of humans in the wake of catastrophe and their relationship with nature and technology. It seems that nature and technology are, for the present-day human being, realms situated externally to ourselves. In the technofix approach, technology is to be used to manipulate nature. Admittedly, in the return-to-nature stance, it seems our proper place is to be part of nature. However, somehow, we have been able to leave nature behind, look at it, and manipulate it from a distance. You could not return to something if you could not leave it in the first place.

In Death Stranding, the world is a hostile but still beautiful place. The apocalyptic landscape is rough, few trees remain, and as a player, one cannot but feel relieved when stumbling upon a small forest or idyllic meadows and creeks. Most of the time, you plough through rocky or even snowy terrain. As for apocalyptic landscapes, Death Stranding sits between the total desolation of *The Road* and the bucolic landscapes of post-apocalyptic movies like *The Quiet Place*, which seem to convey that although the world has ended, we have found our purer, more natural selves. In Death Stranding, human beings' relationship with nature and technology is far more complex. We are on the verge of the sixth mass extinction, which will inevitably include humans and most other-than-human animals. Devastating events have already happened. Technology could not prevent the disasters and may even have caused them. At the same time, technology helps Sam connect the different settlements again, and he can make his journey somewhat more manageable with technology. Nevertheless, he must work with the environment, not against it. If you build too many structures, such as zip lines, resources are saturated, and you must destroy some old ones to make room. Eventually, structures decay under the toxic rain that accelerates time and destruction. When you first venture into new territory, you stumble and fall. I have spent hours climbing snowy hills only to lose my grip and slide down, losing the distance I struggled to gain. But failing is inherent to the game, and reaching the different destinations would have been an altogether different experience if we could straight-on walk there.

Sam is the incarnation of the cyborg figure, as Donna Haraway described in her seminal essay *A Cyborg Manifesto* (Haraway, 1991). This figure challenges the dichotomies that haunt Western thought. It is a boundary figure between organism and machine, man and woman. The cyborg is neither good nor bad. It is not the enemy of humankind, nor is it necessarily its saviour. Sam uses several prosthetic gears, such as exoskeletons, to increase his speed or allow him to carry more weight. At the same time, he has very organic needs, such as urinating and sleeping. His fatigue becomes tangible through the PlayStation controller and sound technology. As a player, you feel your character ploughing through the snow and struggling through tricky waters. When arriving dirty or covered with blood at his shelter, Sam begs you to have him take a shower. Sam Porter Bridges is portrayed by Norman Reedus, a bearded muscular man. He carries with him, on his chest, a pod with an unborn baby. This baby is considered a 'tool' that can warn you when danger is nearby. At the same time, the analogy with pregnancy is obvious: the baby feels Sam's every move, and you can soothe her by playing a song on your harmonica. Sam and the baby gradually grow close, and he eases into a role as her carer.

The reality in which Sam operates is harsh, and the sixth mass extinction is imminent. At the same time, the game has much playfulness, joy, and humour. I am reminded here about the ideas of playfulness by Maria Lugones, whose work I got to know very late in writing this book. As a lesbian of colour in white male-dominated academia, she was told that she was a serious person. However, her friends and family considered her exceptionally playful. When we lose playfulness, we lose a source of wisdom:

> Playfulness is, in part, an openness to being a fool, which is a combination of not worrying about competence, not being self-important, not taking norms as sacred and finding ambiguity and double edges a source of wisdom and delight. (Lugones, 1987)

Death Stranding is not a multiplayer game, but you are connected with other players and see their structures appear in your game world. Some are useful, but some are signs containing hearts and smileys encouraging you to go on. Players send you likes for your constructions, and you can also send them likes. Even your pod baby and the monsters you have to fight can send you likes. The enormous number of likes you can get in the game may be considered a critique of social media addiction or our need for validation and reassurance. At the same time, the likes make the game funny and even light-hearted. It seems that Kojima is telling us that we can only rebuild our world if we do not take ourselves too seriously. Ziplines become available at some point in the game and greatly enhance your efficiency in delivering packages in snowy mountains. The ziplines are sheer joy for Sam, the pod baby, and you, the player, who can almost viscerally experience the giddiness of speeding through the landscape. As Sam, you can pee, provided you have drunk enough water. If you pee on the ghouls, they disappear. Who could blame them? Mushrooms spawn on the spot where you pee, and you can even pee on other players' mushrooms to make bigger ones. If they have been peed on sufficiently, mushrooms become large structures attracting or generating tardigrade-like macroscopic creatures that you can eat to restore vitality. The combination of mushroom, urine, and tardigrade is no coincidence: organic waste is part of the humus that will rebuild the world. To use anthropologist Anna Tsing's words, tardigrades and mushrooms are resilient creatures which can grow in capitalist ruins (Tsing, 2015).

Death Stranding is a shameless and blatant allegory for our near future. The prospect is dire: there are no magic solutions that can stop the inevitable. Nevertheless, it is also a game of hope. It is true that the sixth mass extinction is inevitable and that our time in this universe is limited. Humans are just one episode in the succession of deaths and possibilities that have come and will come with each extinction. However, it may still be worthwhile trying to postpone it, as a character says in the game, 'for a few hundred thousand years'. At the end of the game, America is still in ruins, although people have been reconnected through the Chiral network, a future incarnation of our world wide web. Sam, who does not like company, has made many friends. He has learned to live with the landscape, work with it and enjoy it. The America of Death Stranding is Donna Haraway's Chthulucene, 'a kind of timeplace for learning to stay with the trouble of living and dying in response-ability on a damaged earth' (Haraway, 2016).

Sam stays with the trouble: there is no going back to a time before, no technofix. Instead, as players, we use technology entangled with the possibilities of the landscape, but we must do so responsibly. Sam finds comfort in walking the landscape, jumping over cliffs, ziplining, talking to his baby, and soaking in natural hot springs. We discover what makes humanity worth saving through playing, and it is not necessarily grand ideas. It is joy and connection that inspires responsibility. In the light of total annihilation, seriousness is the biggest vice. For me, the game is an allegory of the heart of bioethics.

Epilogue
Thinking With

In which I leave much to be desired.

If one imagines the We in a circle of its own unity surrounded by circles maintaining their own unity, perhaps the concept of human action as a pebble dropped into a pond would have more meaning. No pebble can be dropped into a pond without its ripples encountering other ripples and those ripples having other consequence through their encounters.

— V. F. Cordova (2003)

 https://doi.org/10.11647/OBP.0320.21

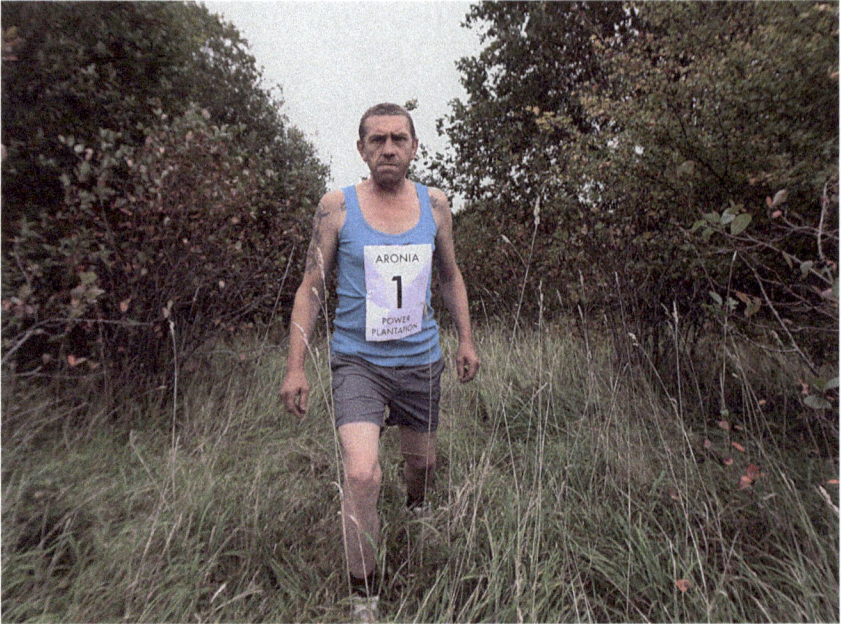

Aroniathon #1: The Grasses are Taking Over.

How to keep the grasses down that overtake the rewilding *Baroa belaobara* (berryapple) plantation.

From: The Aroniathon series.

Model: 'Dzucks'. Photo by Bartaku, 2011[1]

---

1   First photo of the Aroniathon #1 photographic intervention (forty-two photos): a staged, fake marathon with a fake runner´s outfit and a fake marathon runner. Part of Bartaku artistic research instigated by a rewilding *Baroa belaobara* (berryapple) plantation in Aizpute (Lat) between 2009 and 2019, https://bartaku.net/aroniathons/

With this book, I wanted to examine the trouble that is bioethics and reimagine it as an ethics of life. I do not mean solely thinking about ethical questions about life, but instead, I imagine bioethics as a discipline that is inspired by life and cherishes life. That is an acknowledgement that if we, as a human species, want to survive on a damaged planet, we need to think *with* all kinds of life. It means letting go of utopian visions and sterile thought experiments. At the same time, suggesting an ontology on which we can build such bioethics seems blasphemous. That is probably why I, who wrote a traditional PhD on children and biobanks, wanted to be something other than a bioethicist for years. I imagined I could be a philosopher of biology and spend my years thinking about what life is. Alternatively, I could become an anthropologist or sociologist—after all, I love empirical research. At the same time, I realised that bioethicists have the freedom to engage with all these types of research. I came to appreciate and love the grey zone that bioethics occupies between science, medicine, philosophy, and the humanities. In 2022, we face uncertainties and doom scenarios that pandemics and wars bring. For some people, this means that there is no hope for humanity. However, I believe that as 'ethicists of life', bioethicists can contribute to increasing hope. This means widening the scope of bioethics to engage with and perhaps even include environmental ethics and engaging with diversity and experiences. It means being informed by the past and learning to think with the past about possible futures. In dire need, bioethics should be forward-looking and ask what we value, what world can sustain such values, and how we get there.

This approach to bioethics is not new. We could say it was present at the cradle of the discipline, as becomes clear when we revisit Van Rensselaer Potter's book *Bioethics, A Bridge to the Future* (Rensselaer Potter, 1971). Here, he imagines bioethics based on a specific view of biology, with the ultimate goal of preserving humanity. Now, fifty years after the publication of this book, Potter's hope for a new science seems naive. Bioethics, as a discipline, is far removed from the all-encompassing idea he had for it. Even the effects of bioethics on legislation are limited. It would be great if legislators and policymakers would take the survival of the human species as a guiding principle and shared value system in light of significant future uncertainties and dangers. The pandemic has shown us that this is far from the case. Moreover, present-day bioethicists would probably not think that what Potter suggested was related to the current discipline of bioethics. Thinking about a shared value system that spans the entire scope, from individual values and virtues to a worldwide policy, is far removed from our current practice.

Still, I think our field has much to gain if we take some of Potter's ideas, update them, and incorporate them into our practice. However, we also need newer ideas and a fresh look at the task at hand. In this book, I engaged in thinking with many inspiring philosophers and scientists and have wanted to make them relevant to bioethics. I started by describing the idea of philosophy as plumbing, as Mary Midgley used it, and positioned the bioethicist as philosophical plumber par excellence. Bioethicists are often engaged in scientific research projects. They are ideally situated to make the structures and stories explicit to guide a specific scientific practice. Sometimes these structures are weak and need to be fixed. For example, we can question the dualistic nature that is still prevalent in thinking about genes, natures, and environments despite all the scientific evidence to the contrary. Like plumbers dealing with the stench of under-floor soil pipes, bioethicists deal with muddy and messy truths hidden from sight in the world's underbelly. Sterile thought experiments and arguments stripped of their complexity will not do anymore. Besides thinking about structures and dealing head-on with the messiness of the world, bioethicists and plumbers have in common that they connect things. Bioethicists are neither fish nor fowl, and as liminal creatures, they can bind and bring into dialogue disciplines that are usually worlds apart, such as the humanities, biology, and philosophy.

This refreshing relationality is pervasive in many aspects of Mary Midgley's philosophy. She writes about the relationships with other disciplines and the importance of relationships we have with other human beings, other-than-human beings, and the world at large. Such a worldview of connectedness is maybe not so common in Western philosophical thought, but it is deeply entrenched in native philosophies. The Native American philosopher V. F. Cordova describes Native American philosophy and worldview as fundamentally relational. Humans are not atomistic beings but are connected to and in a dynamic relationship with their surroundings, influencing and being influenced. The worldview is reminiscent of process philosophy, a Western concept that has remained somewhat fringe in the philosophical canon but that is gaining more traction lately. Native American philosophy describes the importance of the idea of belonging, of connectedness to a place. Human beings have a specific role to play in their situatedness. They care for places and all creatures belonging there. I think nowadays, our sense of place is cosmopolitan. We are creatures that belong to the whole world, experience the world, and affect the world, and our actions have far-reaching consequences. The Native American idea of caring for places is a powerful metaphor for our relationship and duty to the Earthly ecosystem as a whole. The role of caregivers transcends discussions in environmental ethics about anthropocentrism and ecocentrism and gives human beings a specific task as specific organisms in the ecosystem.

It strikes me as significant that in 21st-century scientific practice, the idea of the interconnectedness of humans and other-than-human organisms such as animals, plants, mushrooms, and bacteria is vindicated. Acknowledging this is, in my view, also recognising that we must keep these connections in mind if we want a liveable future. As demonstrated by epigenetics, but even more by recent findings in microbiology and mycology, the entanglement of all living beings should give us pause as to how bioethics should never be solely about humans and their survival. Indeed, new visions of biology show how playfulness, creativity and chance encounters have been part of life since its earliest beginnings. Creativity should be integral to scientists' and philosophers' methodology if we want to continue living in a liveable world. Bioethicists, as ethicists of life, can play an important role. Life itself can inspire us with joy and the possibility of imagining the future we would like to have. We can help make that future happen by thinking with trouble and insisting on hopeful discourses and routes. Such a feat is not something one discipline can do alone. Bioethics as interdisciplinary is a truism, but I hope to have given the idea of interdisciplinarity some substance. We can playfully engage with colleagues from many different fields, not as competitors or handmaidens, but thinking with them about the world and its future.

Bibliography

Acosta, A. (2012) *Buen Vivir Sumak Kawsay: Una oportunidad para imaginar otros mundos*. Editorial Abya-Yala.

Agar, N. (2008) *Liberal Eugenics: In Defence of Human Enhancement*. John Wiley & Sons.

Ahmed, E. and Hens, K. (2021) "Microbiome in Precision Psychiatry: An Overview of the Ethical Challenges Regarding Microbiome Big Data and Microbiome-Based Interventions," *AJOB Neuroscience*, pp. 1–17. https://doi.org/10.1080/21507740.2021.1958096.

American Psychiatric Association (2013) *Diagnostic and Statistical Manual of Mental Disorders (DSM-5®)*. American Psychiatric Pub.

Barad, K. (2007) *Meeting the Universe Halfway: Quantum Physics and the Entanglement of Matter and Meaning*. Duke University Press.

Barnes, E. (2016) *The Minority Body: A Theory of Disability*. Oxford University Press.

Bateson, P. P. G. and Martin, P. (2001) *Design for a Life: How Biology and Psychology Shape Human Behavior*. Simon and Schuster.

Beauchamp, T. L. and Childress, J. F. (1979) *Principles of Biomedical Ethics*. Oxford University Press.

Beck, U., Lash, S. and Wynne, B. (1992) *Risk Society: Towards a New Modernity*. Sage.

de la Bellacasa, M. P. (2017) *Matters of Care: Speculative Ethics in More Than Human Worlds*. University of Minnesota Press.

Benatar, D. (2008) *Better Never to Have Been: The Harm of Coming Into Existence*. Oxford University Press.

Berger, J. (2009) *Why Look at Animals?* London: Penguin.

Biddle, J. B. and Kukla, R. (2017) "The geography of epistemic risk," *Exploring Inductive Risk: Case Studies of Values in Science*. Oxford University Press, pp. 215–235.

Boden, D. and Chan, S. (2022) "Rethinking the Posthuman in Bioethics," in *Bioethics and the Posthumanities*. 1st ed. Routledge, pp. 25–40. https://doi.org/10.4324/9781003020707-4.

Boorse, C. (1975) "On the Distinction between Disease and Illness," *Philosophy & Public Affairs*. Wiley, 5(1), pp. 49–68. http://www.jstor.org/stable/2265020.

Boorse, C. (1977) "Health as a Theoretical Concept," *Philosophy of Science*, 44(4), pp. 542–573.

Boorse, C. (1997) "A Rebuttal on Health," in *Biomedical Ethics Reviews*. Totowa, NJ: Humana Press, pp. 1–134. https://doi.org/10.1007/978-1-59259-451-1_1.

Borinskaya, S. A., Ermolaev, A. I. and Kolchinsky, E. I. (2019) "Lysenkoism Against Genetics: The Meeting of the Lenin All-Union Academy of Agricultural Sciences of August 1948, Its Background, Causes, and Aftermath," *Genetics*, 212(1), pp. 1–12. https://doi.org/10.1534/genetics.118.301413.

Bosman, A. M. T. (2017) "Disorders Are Reduced Normativity Emerging from the Relationship Between Organisms and Their Environment," in *Parental Responsibility in the Context of Neuroscience and Genetics*. Springer, Cham (International Library of Ethics, Law, and the New Medicine), pp. 35–54. https://link.springer.com/chapter/10.1007/978-3-319-42834-5_3 (Accessed: April 5, 2018).

Bostrom, N. (2005) "In defense of posthuman dignity," *Bioethics*, 19(3), pp. 202–214. https://doi.org/10.1111/j.1467-8519.2005.00437.x.

Bostrom, N. and Ord, T. (2006) "The Reversal Test: Eliminating Status Quo Bias in Applied Ethics," *Ethics*, 116(4), pp. 656–679. https://doi.org/10.1086/505233.

Bråbäck, L. *et al.* (2018) "Childhood Asthma and Smoking Exposures before Conception: A Three-Generational Cohort Study," *Pediatric allergy and immunology: official publication of the European Society of Pediatric Allergy and Immunology*, 29(4), pp. 361–368. https://doi.org/10.1111/pai.12883.

Bretz, T. H. (2020) "Discussing Harm Without Harming," *Environmental ethics*, 42(2), pp. 169–187. https://doi.org/10.5840/enviroethics2020111615.

Canguilhem, G. (1989) *The normal and the pathological*. New York: Zone Books.

Canguilhem, G. (2008) *Knowledge of Life*. Fordham University Press. https://books.google.be/books?id=_LXhae-qDscC.

Caplan, A. (2017) "Promise of orld's first head transplant is truly fake news," *Chicago Tribune*, 13 December. https://www.chicagotribune.com/opinion/commentary/ct-perspec-head-transplant-ethics-1215-story.html.

Carson, R. (2002) *Silent Spring*. Houghton Mifflin Harcourt.

Chamovitz, D. (2012) *What a Plant Knows: A Field Guide to the Senses*. Farrar, Straus and Giroux.

Ciurria, M. (2019) *An Intersectional Feminist Theory of Moral Responsibility*. Taylor & Francis Group.

Clare, E. (2017) *Brilliant Imperfection: Grappling with Cure*. Duke University Press.

Cobb, J. B. and Jr. (2015) *Whitehead Word Book: A Glossary with Alphabetical Index to Technical Terms in Process and Reality*. Process Century Press.

Cooper, R. (2002) "Disease," *Studies in History and Philosophy of Science Part C: Studies in History and Philosophy of Biological and Biomedical Sciences*. Elsevier, 33(2), pp. 263–282. https://doi.org/10.1016/S0039-3681(02)00018-3.

Cordova, V. F. (2003) "Ethics: The We and the I," in Waters, A. (ed.) *American Indian Thought. Philosophical Essays*. Hoboken: Wiley-Blackwell, pp. 173–181.

Cordova, V. F. (2007) *How it is: The Native American Philosophy of V.F. Cordova*. University of Arizona Press.

Creighton, H. and Waddington, C. H. (1958) "The Strategy of the Genes," *AIBS Bulletin*, 8(2), p. 49. https://doi.org/10.2307/1291959.

Cross, C. L. (2018) "Ecofeminism and an Ethic of Care: Developing an Eco-jurisprudence," *AA: l'architecture d'aujourd'hui*, 50(1), pp. 28–40. https://doi.org/10.18820/24150479/aa50i1.2.

Daston, L. (2019) *Against Nature*. MIT Press.

Dawkins, R. (2016) *The Selfish Gene*. Oxford University Press.

Daxinger, L. and Whitelaw, E. (2010) "Transgenerational Epigenetic Inheritance: More Questions than Answers," *Genome Research*, 20(12), pp. 1623–1628. https://doi.org/10.1101/gr.106138.110.

De Block, A., Delaere, P. and Hens, K. (2022) "Philosophy of Science Can Prevent Manslaughter," *Journal of Bioethical Inquiry*. Springer Science and Business Media LLC. https://doi.org/10.1007/s11673-022-10198-4.

De Vreese, L. (2017) "How to Proceed in the Disease Concept Debate? A Pragmatic Approach," *The Journal of Medicine and Philosophy*, 42(4), pp. 424–446. https://doi.org/10.1093/jmp/jhx011.

Dehue, T. (2014) *Betere mensen: over gezondheid als keuze en koopwaar*. Atlas Contact, Uitgeverij.

Del Savio, L., Loi, M. and Stupka, E. (2015) "Epigenetics and Future Generations," *Bioethics*, 29(8), pp. 580–587. https://doi.org/10.1111/bioe.12150.

Despret, V. (2016) *What Would Animals Say if We Asked the Right Questions?* University of Minnesota Press.

Di Paolo, E. A. and De Jaegher, H. (2021) "Enactive Ethics: Difference Becoming Participation," *Topoi. An International Review of Philosophy*. https://doi.org/10.1007/s11245-021-09766-x.

Dias, B. G. and Ressler, K. J. (2014) "Parental Olfactory Experience Influences Behavior and Neural Structure in Subsequent Generations," *Nature Neuroscience*, 17(1), pp. 89–96. https://doi.org/10.1038/nn.3594.

Dobson, A. P. *et al.* (2020) "Ecology and Economics for Pandemic Prevention," *Science*, 369(6502), pp. 379–381. https://doi.org/10.1126/science.abc3189.

Douglas, H. (2000) "Inductive Risk and Values in Science," *Philosophy of Science*, 67(4), pp. 559–579. https://doi.org/10.1086/392855.

Dugatkin, L. A. and Trut, L. (2017) *How to Tame a Fox (and Build a Dog): Visionary Scientists and a Siberian Tale of Jump-Started Evolution*. University of Chicago Press.

Dupras, C., Saulnier, K. M. and Joly, Y. (2019) "Epigenetics, Ethics, Law and Society: A Multidisciplinary Review of Descriptive, Instrumental, Dialectical and Reflexive Analyses," *Social Studies of Science*, 49(5), pp. 785–810. https://doi.org/10.1177/0306312719866007.

Elliott, C. (1999) *A Philosophical Disease: Bioethics, Culture, and Identity*. Psychology Press.

Francione, G. (2012) *Animals, Property & The Law*. Temple University Press.

Frégnac, Y. and Laurent, G. (2014) *Neuroscience: Where is the brain in the Human Brain Project?* https://doi.org/10.1038/513027a.

Fresco, L. O. (2021) *De plantenjager uit Leningrad*. Prometheus.

Fricker, M. (2009) *Epistemic Injustice: Power and the Ethics of Knowing*. Oxford University Press.

Fukuyama, F. (2002) *Our Posthuman Future: Consequences of the Biotechnology Revolution*. 1st ed. New York: Farrar, Straus and Giroux.

Galton, F. (1895) *English Men of Science: Their Nature and Nurture*. D. Appleton.

Garland-Thomson, R. (2012) "The Case for Conserving Disability," *Journal of Bioethical Inquiry*. Springer Verlag, 9(3), pp. 339–355. https://doi.org/10.1007/s11673-012-9380-0.

Gilbert, S. F. (2015) *Ecological Developmental Biology*. Sinauer.

Gilligan, C. (1982) *In a Different Voice: Psychological Theory and Women's Development*. Harvard University Press.

Giroux, E. (2019) "The Individual Relativity of Health and Disease: Personalized Medicine in the Light of Canguilhem's Philosophy of Medicine." https://www.academia.edu/40407055/The_Individual_Relativity_of_Health_and_Disease_Personalized_Medicine_in_the_Light_of_Canguilhems_Philosophy_of_Medicine.

Grosz, E. (2011) *Becoming Undone: Darwinian Reflections on Life, Politics, and Art*. Duke University Press.

Guerrero-Bosagna, C. (2016) "High Type II Error and Interpretation Inconsistencies when Attempting to Refute Transgenerational Epigenetic Inheritance," *Genome Biology*, 17, p. 153. https://doi.org/10.1186/s13059-016-0982-4.

Hacking, I. (1996) "The Looping Effects of Human Kinds," in Sperber, D., Premack, D., and Premack, A. J. (eds) *Causal Cognition*. Oxford University Press, pp. 351–383.

Hacking, I. (2000) *The Social Construction of What?* Harvard University Press.

Hacking, I. (2004) *Historical Ontology*. Harvard University Press.

Hacking, I. (2009) "Humans, Aliens & Autism," *Daedalus*, 138(3), pp. 44–59. https://doi.org/10.1162/daed.2009.138.3.44.

Hacking, I. (2010) "How We Have Been Learning to Talk About Autism: A Role for Stories," in Kittay, E. F. and Carlson, L. (eds) *Cognitive Disability and Its Challenge to Moral Philosophy*. Wiley-Blackwell, pp. 260–278. https://doi.org/10.1002/9781444322781.ch15.

Haraway, D. (1988) "Situated Knowledges: The Science Question in Feminism and the Privilege of Partial Perspective," *Feminist studies: FS*, 14(3), pp. 575–599. https://doi.org/10.2307/3178066.

Haraway, D. (1991) "A Cyborg Manifesto: Science, Technology, and Socialist-Feminism in the Late Twentieth Century," in *Simians, Cyborgs and Women: The Reinvention of Nature*. Routledge, pp. 149–181.

Haraway, D. J. (1997) *Modest−Witness@Second−Millennium.FemaleMan−Meets−OncoMouse: Feminism and Technoscience*. Psychology Press.

Haraway, D. J. (2007) *The Companion Species Manifesto: Dogs, People, and Significant Otherness*. Prickly Paradigm Press.

Haraway, D. J. (2013) *When Species Meet*. University of Minnesota Press.

Haraway, D. J. (2016) *Staying with the Trouble: Making Kin in the Chthulucene*. Duke University Press.

Harding, S. (1991) *Whose Science? Whose Knowledge?: Thinking from Women's Lives*. Cornell University Press.

Harding, S. (1995) "'Strong objectivity': A Response to the New Objectivity Question," *Synthese*, 104(3), pp. 331–349. https://doi.org/10.1007/BF01064504.

Harris, J. (2005) "Reproductive Liberty, Disease and Disability," *Reproductive biomedicine online*, 10, pp. 13–16. https://doi.org/10.1016/s1472-6483(10)62197-9.

ten Have, H. A. M. J. (2019) *Wounded Planet: How Declining Biodiversity Endangers Health and How Bioethics Can Help*. JHU Press.

ten Have, H. A. M. J. (2022) *Bizarre Bioethics: Ghosts, Monsters, and Pilgrims*. Johns Hopkins University Press.

Hens, K. (2009) "Ethical Responsibilities Towards Dogs: An Inquiry into the Dog–Human Relationship," *Journal of Agricultural & Environmental Ethics*, 22(1), pp. 3–14. https://doi.org/10.1007/s10806-008-9120-y.

Hens, K. *et al.* (2019) "Blurring Boundaries. Interviews With PGT Couples About Comprehensive Chromosome Screening," *European Journal of Medical Genetics*, 62(12), p. 103604. https://doi.org/10.1016/j.ejmg.2018.12.009.

Hens, K. (2017) "The Ethics of Postponed Fatherhood," *IJFAB: International Journal of Feminist Approaches to Bioethics*, 10(1), pp. 103–118. https://doi.org/10.3138/ijfab.10.1.103.

Hens, K. (2021) *Towards an Ethics of Autism*. Open Book Publishers. https://doi.org/10.11647/OBP.0261.

Hens, K., Dondorp, W. and de Wert, G. (2015) "A Leap of Faith? An Interview Study With Professionals on the Use of Mitochondrial Replacement to Avoid Transfer of Mitochondrial Diseases," *Human Reproduction*, 30(5), pp. 1256–1262. https://doi.org/10.1093/humrep/dev056.

Hens, K. and Langenberg, R. (2018) *Experiences of Adults Following an Autism Diagnosis*. Springer International Publishing.

Hens, K., Peeters, H. and Dierickx, K. (2016a) "Genetic Testing and Counseling in the Case of an Autism Diagnosis: A Caregivers Perspective," *European Journal of Medical Genetics*, 59(9), pp. 452–458. https://doi.org/10.1016/j.ejmg.2016.08.007.

Hens, K., Peeters, H. and Dierickx, K. (2016b) "Shooting a Moving Target. Researching Autism Genes: An Interview Study with Professionals," *European Journal of Medical Genetics*, 59(1), pp. 32–38. https://doi.org/10.1016/j.ejmg.2015.12.009.

Houri-Zeevi, L. *et al.* (2021) "Stress resets Ancestral Heritable Small RNA Responses," *eLife*, 10. https://doi.org/10.7554/eLife.65797.

Hummer, R. A. and Hernandez, E. M. (2013) "The Effect of Educational Attainment on Adult Mortality in the United States," *Population bulletin*, 68(1), pp. 1–16. https://www.ncbi.nlm.nih.gov/pubmed/25995521.

IJFAB: International Journal of Feminist Approaches to Bioethics (no date). https://www.ijfab.org/

Jablonka, E. (2016) "Cultural Epigenetics," *The Sociological Review*, 64(1_suppl), pp. 42–60. https://doi.org/10.1111/2059-7932.12012.

Jablonka, E. and Lamb, M. J. (2014) *Evolution in Four Dimensions, revised edition: Genetic, Epigenetic, Behavioral, and Symbolic Variation in the History of Life*. MIT Press.

Johannsen, W. (1911) "The Genotype Conception of Heredity," *The American Naturalist*, 45(531), pp. 129–159.

Johnston, T. D. (1987) "The Persistence of Dichotomies in the Study of Behavioral Development," *Developmental Review: DR*, 7(2), pp. 149–182. https://doi.org/10.1016/0273-2297(87)90011-6.

Jones, K. E. *et al.* (2008) "Global Trends in Emerging Infectious Diseases," *Nature*, 451(7181), pp. 990–993. https://doi.org/10.1038/nature06536.

Juengst, E. T. *et al.* (2014) "Serving Epigenetics Before its Time," *Trends in genetics: TIG*, 30(10), pp. 427–429. https://doi.org/10.1016/j.tig.2014.08.001.

Kafer, A. (2013) *Feminist, Queer, Crip*. Indiana University Press.

Kauffman, S. A. (2016) *Humanity in a Creative Universe*. Oxford University Press.

Kauffman, S. A. (2019) *A World Beyond Physics: The Emergence and Evolution of Life*. Oxford University Press.

Kauffman, S. A. (1993) *The Origins of Order: Self-organization and Selection in Evolution*. Oxford University Press.

Keeling, D. M. and Lehman, M. N. (2018) "Posthumanism," in *Oxford Research Encyclopedia of Communication*. https://doi.org/10.1093/acrefore/9780190228613.013.627.

Keller, E. F. (2010) *The Mirage of a Space between Nature and Nurture*. Duke University Press.

Kittay, E. F. (2019) *Learning from My Daughter: The Value and Care of Disabled Minds*. Oxford University Press.

Klosin, A. *et al.* (2017) "Transgenerational Transmission of Environmental Information in C. Elegans," *Science*, 356(6335), pp. 320–323. https://doi.org/10.1126/science.aah6412.

Kopnina, H. *et al.* (2018) "Anthropocentrism: More than Just a Misunderstood Problem," *Journal of agricultural & Environmental Ethics*, 31(1), pp. 109–127. https://doi.org/10.1007/s10806-018-9711-1.

Krenak, A. (2020) *Ideas to Postpone the End of the World*. House of Anansi Press Incorporated.

Kvaale, E. P., Haslam, N. and Gottdiener, W. H. (2013) "The 'Side Effects' of Medicalization: A Meta-Analytic Review of How Biogenetic Explanations Affect Stigma," *Clinical Psychology Review*, 33(6), pp. 782–794. https://doi.org/10.1016/j.cpr.2013.06.002.

Lehrman, D. S. (1953) "A Critique of Konrad Lorenz's Theory of Instinctive Behavior," *The Quarterly Review of Biology*, 28(4), pp. 337–363. https://doi.org/10.1086/399858.

Levin, K. *et al.* (2012) "Overcoming The Tragedy of Super Wicked Problems: Constraining our Future Selves to Ameliorate Global Climate Change," *Policy Sciences*, 45(2), pp. 123–152. https://doi.org/10.1007/s11077-012-9151-0.

Lindemann, H. (2006) *An Invitation to Feminist Ethics*. McGraw-Hill.

Lindemann, H., Verkerk, M. and Walker, M. U. (2008) *Naturalized Bioethics: Toward Responsible Knowing and Practice*. Cambridge University Press..

Linett, M. T. (2020) *Literary Bioethics: Animality, Disability, and the Human*. New York University Press.

Longo, G., Montévil, M. and Kauffman, S. (2012) "No Entailing Laws, but Enablement in the Evolution of the Biosphere," in *Proceedings of the 14th Annual Conference Companion on Genetic and Evolutionary Computation*. New York: Association for Computing Machinery (GECCO '12), pp. 1379–1392. https://doi.org/10.1145/2330784.2330946.

Lugones, M. (1987) "Playfulness, 'World'-Travelling, and Loving Perception," *Hypatia*, 2(2), pp. 3–19.

Ma, Y. *et al.* (2018) "Help, Hope and Hype: Ethical Considerations of Human Microbiome Research and Applications," *Protein & Cell*, 9(5), pp. 404–415. https://doi.org/10.1007/s13238-018-0537-4.

Maienschein, J. (2000) "Competing Epistemologies and Developmental Biology," in Creath, R. and Maienschein, J. (eds) *Biology and Epistemology*. Cambridge University Press, pp. 122–137. https://philpapers.org/rec/MAICEA.

Margulis, L. (2008) *Symbiotic Planet: A New Look At Evolution*. Basic Books.

Meloni, M. (2016) *Political Biology: Science and Social Values in Human Heredity from Eugenics to Epigenetics*. Springer.

Midgley, M. (1992) "Philosophical Plumbing," *Royal Institute of Philosophy Supplement*, 33, pp. 139–151. https://doi.org/10.1017/S1358246100002319.

Midgley, M. (2004) *The Myths We Live by*. Psychology Press.

Midgley, M. (2018) *What Is Philosophy for?* Bloomsbury Publishing.

Mills, Charles W. and Mills, Charles Wade (1997) *The Racial Contract*. Cornell University Press.

Millum, J. and Emanuel, E. J. (2012) *Global Justice and Bioethics*. Oxford University Press.

Money, N. P. (2021) *Nature Fast and Nature Slow: How Life Works, from Fractions of a Second to Billions of Years*. Reaktion Books.

Moore, D. S. (2003) *The Dependent Gene: The Fallacy of "Nature Vs. Nurture."* Henry Holt & Co.

Moore, G. E. (1993) *Principia Ethica*. Cambridge University Press.

More, M. (1994) "On Becoming Posthuman," *Free inquiry*, 14(4), pp. 38–41. https://philpapers.org/rec/MOROBP.

Morgan, T. H. (1910) "Sex Limited Inheritance in Drosophila," *Science*, 32(812), pp. 120–122. https://doi.org/10.1126/science.32.812.120.

Murphy, D. (2021) "Concepts of Disease and Health," *The Stanford Encyclopedia of Philosophy*. Spring. Edited by E. N. Zalta. Metaphysics Research Lab, Stanford University. https://plato.stanford.edu/archives/spr2021/entries/health-disease/.

Naess, A. (1986) "The Deep Ecological Movement: Some Philosophical Aspects," *Philosophical Inquiry*, 8(1/2), pp. 10–31. https://doi.org/10.5840/philinquiry198681/22.

Nakamura, M. *et al.* (2021) "CRISPR Technologies for Precise Epigenome Editing," *Nature Cell Biology*, 23(1), pp. 11–22. https://doi.org/10.1038/s41556-020-00620-7.

Nelkin, D. and Lindee, M. S. (2004) *The DNA Mystique: The Gene as a Cultural Icon*. University of Michigan.

Noble, D. (2006) *The Music of Life: Biology Beyond the Genome*. Oxford: Oxford University Press.

Ohno, M. and Caughey, A. (2013) "The Role of Noninvasive Prenatal Testing as a Diagnostic Versus a Screening Tool: A Cost-Effectiveness Analysis," *Prenatal Diagnosis*, 33(7), pp. 630–635. https://doi.org/10.1002/pd.4156.

O'Neill, O. (2002) *Autonomy and Trust in Bioethics*. Cambridge University Press.

Oyama, S., Griffiths, P. E. and Gray, R. D. (2003) *Cycles of Contingency: Developmental Systems and Evolution*. MIT Press.

Oyěwùmí, O. (1997) *The Invention of Women: Making an African Sense of Western Gender Discourses*. University of Minnesota Press.

Painter, R. C. *et al.* (2008) "Transgenerational Effects of Prenatal Exposure to the Dutch Famine on Neonatal Adiposity and Health in Later Life," *BJOG: An International Journal of Obstetrics and Gynaecology*, 115(10), pp. 1243–1249. https://doi.org/10.1111/j.1471-0528.2008.01822.x.

Parfit, D. (1984) *Reasons and Persons*. Oxford University Press.

Perroud, N. *et al.* (2014) "The Tutsi Genocide and Transgenerational Transmission of Maternal Stress: Epigenetics and Biology of the HPA Axis," *The World Journal of Biological Psychiatry: The Official Journal of the World Federation of Societies of Biological Psychiatry*, 15(4), pp. 334–345. https://doi.org/10.3109/15622975.2013.866693.

Phelan, J. C. (2005) "Geneticization of Deviant Behavior and Consequences for Stigma: The Case of Mental Illness," *Journal of Health and Social Behavior*. 46(4), pp. 307–322. https://doi.org/10.1177/002214650504600401.

Plumwood, V. (2012) *The Eye of the Crocodile*. ANU E Press.

Potter, V. R. (1988) *Global Bioethics: Building on the Leopold Legacy*. Michigan State University Press.

Pozzer, A. *et al.* (2020) "Regional and Global Contributions of air Pollution to Risk of Death From COVID-19," *Cardiovascular Research*, 116(14), pp. 2247–2253. https://doi.org/10.1093/cvr/cvaa288.

Prigogine, I. V. and Stengers, I. (1984) *Order Out of Chaos: Man's New Dialogue with Nature*. Bantam Books.

Prigogine, I. and Stengers, I. (1997) *The End of Certainty*. Simon and Schuster.

Railton, P. (1986) "Moral Realism," *The Philosophical Review*. Duke University Press, 95(2), pp. 163–207. https://doi.org/10.2307/2185589.

Rawls, J. (1999) *A Theory of Justice*. Rev. ed. Belknap Press of Harvard University Press.

Reardon, J. *et al.* (2015) "Science & Justice: The Trouble and the Promise," *Catalyst: Feminism, Theory, Technoscience*, 1(1), pp. 1–49. https://doi.org/10.28968/cftt.v1i1.28817.

Rensselaer Potter, V. (1971) *Bioethics: Bridge to the Future*. Prentice-Hall.

Rhodes, R. (2016) "Ethical Issues in Microbiome Research and Medicine," *BMC Medicine*, 14(1), p. 156. https://doi.org/10.1186/s12916-016-0702-7.

Richards, R. J. (1974) "The Innate and the Learned: The Evolution of Konrad Lorenz's Theory of Instinct," *Philosophy of the Social Sciences*, 4(2–3), pp. 111–133. https://doi.org/10.1177/004839317400400201.

Richerson, P. J. and Boyd, R. (2006) *Not by Genes Alone: How Culture Transformed Human Evolution*. 1st ed. University of Chicago Press.

Richie, C. (2019) *Principles of Green Bioethics: Sustainability in Health Care*. Michigan State University Press.

Robles-Matos, N. *et al.* (2021) "Environmental Exposure to Endocrine Disrupting Chemicals Influences Genomic Imprinting, Growth, and Metabolism," *Genes*, 12(8). https://doi.org/10.3390/genes12081153.

Rockström, J. *et al.* (2009) "A safe operating space for humanity," *Nature*, 461(7263), pp. 472–475. https://doi.org/10.1038/461472a.

Rogers, W. A. *et al.* (2022) *The Routledge Handbook of Feminist Bioethics*. Taylor & Francis.

Roy, M.-C., Dupras, C. and Ravitsky, V. (2017) "The Epigenetic Effects of Assisted Reproductive Technologies: Ethical Considerations," *Journal of Developmental Origins of Health and Disease*, 8(4), pp. 436–442. https://doi.org/10.1017/S2040174417000344.

Russell, W. M. S. and Burch, R. L. (1959) *The Principles of Humane Experimental Technique*. Methuen.

Sands, D. (2022) *Bioethics and the Posthumanities*. Routledge.

Santaló, J. and Berdasco, M. (2022) "Ethical Implications of Epigenetics in the Era of Personalized Medicine," *Clinical Epigenetics*, 14(1), p. 44. https://doi.org/10.1186/s13148-022-01263-1.

Savulescu, J. (2001) "Procreative beneficence: why we should select the best children," *Bioethics*, 15(5–6), pp. 413–426. https://www.ncbi.nlm.nih.gov/pubmed/12058767.

Savulescu, J. and Kahane, G. (2009) "The moral obligation to create children with the best chance of the best life," *Bioethics*, 23, pp. 274–290. https://doi.org/10.1111/j.1467-8519.2008.00687.x.

Schaffner, K. F. (2016) *Behaving: What's Genetic, What's Not, and why Should We Care?* Oxford University Press.

Schaubroeck, K. and Hens, K. (2021) "Pandemic Risk and Standpoint Epistemology: A Matter of Solidarity," *Health Care Analysis: HCA: Journal of Health Philosophy and Policy*. https://doi.org/10.1007/s10728-021-00443-z.

Schick, A. (2016) "Whereto speculative bioethics? Technological visions and future simulations in a science fictional culture," *Medical humanities*, 42(4), pp. 225–231. https://doi.org/10.1136/medhum-2016-010951.

Scully, J. L. (2008) *Disability Bioethics: Moral Bodies, Moral Difference*. Rowman & Littlefield.

Scully, J. L. (2012) "The Convention on the Rights of Persons with Disabilities and Cultural Understandings of Disability," in Anderson, J. and Philips, J. (eds) *Disability and Universal Human Rights: Legal, Ethical and Conceptual Implications of the Convention on the Rights of Persons with Disabilities*. Utrecht: Netherlands Institute of Human Rights (SIM), pp. 71–83.

Sgreccia, E. (2012) *Personalist Bioethics: Foundations and Applications*. National Catholic Bioethics Center.

Sheldrake, M. (2021) *Entangled Life: How Fungi Make Our Worlds, Change Our Minds & Shape Our Futures*. Random House Publishing Group.

Shepard, P. (1997) *The Others: How Animals Made Us Human*. Island Press.

Skarsaune, S. N., Hanisch, H. and Gjermestad, A. (2021) "Self-Determination: What can we Learn from Persons with Profound Intellectual and Multiple Disabilities?," *Scandinavian Journal of Disability Research: SJDR*. Stockholm University Press, 23(1), pp. 317–327. https://doi.org/10.16993/sjdr.830.

Skinner, M. K. (2014) "Environmental Stress and Epigenetic Transgenerational Inheritance," *BMC Medicine*, 12, p. 153. https://doi.org/10.1186/s12916-014-0153-y.

Snow, C. P. (1993) *The Two Cultures*. Cambridge University Press.

Solnit, R. (2016) *Hope in the Dark: Untold Histories, Wild Possibilities*. Haymarket Books.

Spiel, K. and Gerling, K. (2020) "The Purpose of Play: How HCI Games Research Fails Neurodivergent Populations," *ACM Trans. Comput.-Hum. Interact.*, 1(1).

Stegenga, J. (2018) *Medical Nihilism*. Oxford University Press.

Steinbock, B. (1992) *Life Before Birth: The Moral and Legal Status of Embryos and Fetuses: The Moral and Legal Status of Embryos and Fetuses*. Oxford University Press.

Stengers, I. (2005) "The Cosmopolitical Proposal," in Latour, B. and Weibel, P. (eds) *Making Things Public*. MIT Press, pp. 994–1003. https://philpapers. org/rec/STETCP-4.

Stengers, I. (2020) *Réactiver le sens commun: Lecture de Whitehead en temps de débâcle*. La Découverte.

Stramondo, J. A. (2021) "Tragic Choices: Disability, Triage, and Equity Amidst a Global Pandemic," *Journal of Philosophy of Disability*, 1, pp. 201–210. https:// doi.org/10.5840/jpd20219206.

Strugatsky, A., Strugatsky, B. and Bormashenko, O. (2012) *Roadside Picnic*. Chicago Review Press.

Tavory, I., Jablonka, E. and Ginsburg, S. (2014) "The reproduction of the social: a developmental system theory approach," in *Scaffolding in Evolution, Culture and Cognition: Vienna Series in Theoretical Biology*. MIT Press, pp. 307–327. https://nyuscholars.nyu.edu/en/publications/ the-reproduction-of-the-social-a-developmental-system-theory-appr.

The Lancet (2020) "Facing up to long COVID," *The Lancet*, 396(10266), p. 1861. https://doi.org/10.1016/S0140-6736(20)32662-3.

Tronto, J. C. (2013) *Caring Democracy: Markets, Equality, and Justice*. New York University Press.

Tsing, A. L. (2015) *The Mushroom at the End of the World: On the Possibility of Life in Capitalist Ruins*. Princeton University Press.

Tsing, A. L. *et al.* (2017) *Arts of Living on a Damaged Planet: Ghosts of the Anthropocene*. University of Minnesota Press.

Tuan, Y.-F. (1984) *Dominance & Affection: The Making of Pets*. Yale University Press.

Van Dooren, T. (2019) *The Wake of Crows: Living and Dying in Shared Worlds*. Columbia University Press.

Van Goidsenhoven, L. and De Schauwer, E. (2020) "Listening beyond words: Swinging together," *Scandinavian Journal of Disability Research: SJDR*. Stockholm University Press, 22(1), pp. 330–339. https://doi.org/10.16993/ sjdr.756.

Vanaken (2022) "Cripping vulnerability: A disability bioethics approach to the case of early autism interventions," *Journal for Gender Studies / Tijdschrift voor Genderstudies*. https://doi.org/10.5117/TVGN2022.1.002.VANA.

Varela, F. J., Rosch, E. and Thompson, E. (1992) *The Embodied Mind: Cognitive Science and Human Experience*. MIT Press.

Veldkamp, S. A. M. *et al.* (2019) "Genetic and Environmental Influences on Different Forms of Bullying Perpetration, Bullying Victimization, and Their Co-occurrence," *Behavior Genetics*, 49(5), pp. 432–443. https://doi.org/10.1007/s10519-019-09968-5.

Victor, E. and Guidry-Grimes, L. K. (2021) *Applying Nonideal Theory to Bioethics: Living and Dying in a Nonideal World*. Springer International Publishing.

Waddington, C. H. (1944) *Science and Ethics: An Essay*. G. Allen & Unwin.

Watchmen (2008). Dc Comics.

Wee, M. (2022) "Therapy, Enhancement, and the Social Model of Disability," in *Bioethics and the Posthumanities*. 1st ed. Routledge, pp. 15–24. https://doi.org/10.4324/9781003020707-3.

Wessel, A. (2009) "What is epigenesis? or Gene's Place in Development," *human_ontogenetics*. Wiley, 3(2), pp. 35–37. https://doi.org/10.1002/huon.200900008.

Whitehead, A. N. (1967) *Science and the Modern World*. Simon and Schuster.

Whitehead, A. N. (2010) *Process and Reality*. Simon and Schuster.

Whitehead, A. N. and Price, L. (2001) *Dialogues of Alfred North Whitehead*. David R. Godine Publisher.

Whitehead, A. N. and Russell, B. (1927) *Principia Mathematica*. Cambridge University Press.

Whitelaw, E. (2015) "Disputing Lamarckian epigenetic inheritance in mammals," *Genome biology*, 16, p. 60. https://doi.org/10.1186/s13059-015-0626-0.

Whyte, K. and Cuomo, C. J. (2016) "Ethics of Caring in Environmental Ethics: Indigenous and Feminist Philosophies." https://papers.ssrn.com/abstract=2770065 (Accessed: March 9, 2022).

Wieseler, C. (2020) "Epistemic oppression and ableism in bioethics," *Hypatia*, 35(4), pp. 714–732. https://doi.org/10.1017/hyp.2020.38.

Wilson, E. A. (2015) *Gut Feminism*. Duke University Press.

Young, I. M. (2011) *Responsibility for Justice*. Oxford University Press.

Zylinska, J. (2009) *Bioethics in the Age of New Media*. MIT Press.

Index

About the Team

Alessandra Tosi was the managing editor for this book.

Joanne Walton and Lucy Barnes performed the copy-editing and proofreading.

Jeevanjot Nagpal designed the cover. The cover was produced in InDesign using the Fontin font.

Luca Baffa typeset the book in InDesign and produced the paperback and hardback editions. The text font is Tex Gyre Pagella; the heading font is Californian FB.

Luca produced the EPUB, AZW3, PDF, HTML, and XML editions — the conversion is performed with open source software such as pandoc (https://pandoc.org/) created by John MacFarlane and other tools freely available on our GitHub page (https://github.com/OpenBookPublishers).

This book need not end here...

Share

All our books — including the one you have just read — are free to access online so that students, researchers and members of the public who can't afford a printed edition will have access to the same ideas. This title will be accessed online by hundreds of readers each month across the globe: why not share the link so that someone you know is one of them?

This book and additional content is available at:

https://doi.org/10.11647/OBP.0320

Donate

Open Book Publishers is an award-winning, scholar-led, not-for-profit press making knowledge freely available one book at a time. We don't charge authors to publish with us: instead, our work is supported by our library members and by donations from people who believe that research shouldn't be locked behind paywalls.

Why not join them in freeing knowledge by supporting us: https://www.openbookpublishers.com/support-us

Follow @OpenBookPublish 🐦

Read more at the Open Book Publishers **BLOG**

You may also be interested in:

Towards an Ethics of Autism
A Philosophical Exploration
Kristien Hens

https://doi.org/10.11647/OBP.0261

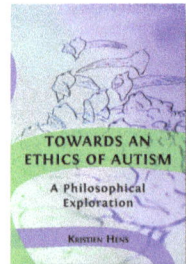

Foundations for Moral Relativism
Second Expanded Edition
J. David Velleman

https://doi.org/10.11647/OBP.0086

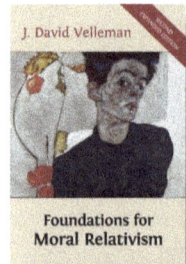

Human Cultures through the Scientific Lens
Essays in Evolutionary Cognitive Anthropology
Pascal Boyer

https://doi.org/10.11647/OBP.0257

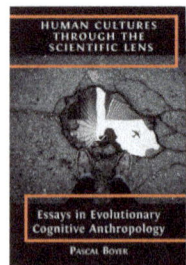